Journal Article

Writing

and

Publication

Your Guide to Mastering Clinical Health Care Reporting Standards

Journal Article

Writing

and

Publication

Your Guide to Mastering Clinical Health Care Reporting Standards

Sharon A. Gutman, PhD, OTR, FAOTA

Associate Professor of Rehabilitation and Regenerative Medicine
Columbia University Medical Center
Programs in Occupational Therapy
New York, New York

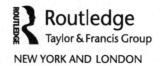

Routledge
Taylor & Francis Group

NEW YORK AND LONDON

First published in 2017 SLACK Incorporated

Published 2024 by Routledge
605 Third Avenue, New York, NY 10058

and by Routledge
4 Park Square, Milton Park, Abingdon, Oxon OX14 4RN

Routledge is an imprint of the Taylor & Francis Group, an informa business

© 2017 Taylor & Francis Group

Dr. Sharon A. Gutman has no financial or proprietary interest in the materials presented herein.

Library of Congress Cataloging-in-Publication Data

Names: Gutman, Sharon A., author.
Title: Journal article writing and publication : your guide to mastering
  clinical health care reporting standards / Sharon A. Gutman.
Description: Thorofare, NJ : Slack Incorporated, [2017] | Includes
  bibliographical references and index.
Identifiers: LCCN 2016034966| ISBN 9781630913342 (paperback : alk. paper) |
Subjects: | MESH: Medical Writing--standards | Health Services
  Research--standards | Manuscripts as Topic | Periodicals as
  Topic--standards | Authorship--standards
Classification: LCC R119 | NLM WZ 345 | DDC 808.06/661--dc23 LC record available at
https://lccn.loc.gov/2016034966

ISBN: 9781630913342 (pbk)
ISBN: 9781003524717 (ebk)

DOI: 10.4324/9781003524717

Contents

Acknowledgments

I thank Dr. Jane Case-Smith and Dr. Rondalyn Whitney for help with the conceptualization of this book. I also thank Dr. Janet Falk-Kessler for sharing our article, "Development and Psychometric Properties of the Emotional Intelligence Admission Essay Scale," in Chapter 9.

About the Author

Sharon A. Gutman, PhD, OTR, FAOTA is an occupational therapist and associate professor at Columbia University Medical Center. In a career spanning 25 years, she has published 42 peer-reviewed articles, 7 textbooks, 6 textbook chapters, 24 editorials as editor-in-chief of the *American Journal of Occupational Therapy* (*AJOT*), and 5 continuing education articles and courses. Dr. Gutman served as the editor-in-chief of *AJOT* between 2008 and 2014, during which time she helped practitioners and researchers better understand manuscript writing, clinical study reporting standards, intervention fidelity, research methodologies, health literacy, and copyright issues. A major initiative of her editorship was to help researchers better understand the need for evidence-based research to support health care practice and the design and implementation of intervention effectiveness studies. By the end of her *AJOT* editorship, she had increased the publication of clinical intervention studies by 50% and helped to increase the journal impact factor score from an average of 0.641 over a 10-year period (1998–2007) to a 5-year score of 2.021 in 2014. In this book Dr. Gutman summarizes her 25 years of experience and knowledge to help students and researchers better understand the use of health care reporting standards in manuscript preparation, the reporting of statistical data in text, and the manuscript review and revision process. Readers will find this book easy to use and critical to a successful writing career in academia and research.

1

Introduction
The Importance of Writing to
Advance Your Career and Profession

Health care professions have an implicit contract with society to provide services that are effective and cost-efficient. Until recently, however, health care professions were not held accountable by society to demonstrate clinical effectiveness. Although the Food and Drug Administration has for years required a rigorous protocol for pharmaceutical and medical device testing (U.S. Department of Health and Human Services, 2015), this same demand for accountability of service has not been required of most health care practices. Managed care's denial of reimbursement for new, experimental, and unproven interventions has largely been the impetus for health care researchers to demonstrate the effectiveness of treatment. Increased health care litigation and malpractice costs have similarly compelled health care professionals to demonstrate service effectiveness through empirical research.

The ability to demonstrate that a specific health care profession provides valuable and effective services that meet society's health needs is a major objective for all health care academicians and researchers. Such skills are critical to ensure service reimbursement from an increasingly small pool of health care dollars. Demonstrating clinical effectiveness depends on the ability to obtain funding support for clinical research. Obtaining funding depends on research skills and the ability to convey through writing how a study will contribute to the health of society's members. Grant funding has become critical to obtain the resources needed to implement research that can support the effectiveness of health care practices.

More critical is the reporting of written research results through journal publication so that the health care community and larger society will be able to access and read evidence supporting health care services. Good writing skills, however, are not sufficient for journal publication. Today, several clinical reporting standard guidelines have been created by researchers to enhance the ability of readers to evaluate the quality and value of studies. To my knowledge, this book is a first attempt to compile those clinical research reporting standards in one source. Health care

Gutman, S. A. *Journal Article Writing and Publication:*
Your Guide to Mastering Clinical Health Care Reporting Standards
(pp. 1-3). © 2017 Taylor & Francis Group.

researchers must begin using these reporting standards in order to write manuscripts that are correctly formatted and transparently convey all critical study strengths and limitations. Educators must teach these reporting standards to students, who must evaluate research reports as consumers and who, in the future, may contribute to the literature through their own writing. As a former editor of the *American Journal of Occupational Therapy* (*AJOT*), I can attest that most authors, even seasoned writers, were unaware of these guidelines and needed moderate guidance to reformat their manuscripts in accordance with them.

Learning about and consistently using reporting standards in journal publication is important to the advancement of health care professions. But such advancement begins with our own individual efforts. As of this writing, many health care professions have a shortage of well-prepared educators and researchers. To earn a position in the academy—to be employed as a faculty member in an institution of higher learning—educators must have obtained a research doctoral degree. In most institutions of higher learning, promotion and tenure require a 7-year period of teaching, service, and publication. These have been the traditional measures of success in academia for the last century and will not change. To be accepted as a peer in an academic setting, health care educators must follow the same route of earning a research doctoral degree and contributing to the scientific community through teaching and scholarship. As educators, we must advance our own careers by earning research doctoral degrees and publishing innovative health care studies that can be applied for the good of society. If we want to be respected by our academic peers who hold research doctoral degrees and have grant and publication histories, we must follow the same path. If we want to advance in the academic environment—receive promotion and tenure and participate in important committees making decisions about university governance—we must earn the same credentials and produce the same level of scholarship as our non-health care academic peers. If we want our health care education programs to be securely situated in, valued by, and respected by the university, we must meet and exceed the university's prescribed measures of academic success.

This is not an easy path. Many of us have come to our health professions as practitioners. We graduated from health care programs and practiced for a number of years before earning a doctoral degree. After the awarding of our doctoral degree, we found that positions as educators were plentiful and did not require postdoctoral work or the need for continued income delay, as is traditional in the basic sciences. There was a price to be paid, however, for forgoing the postdoctoral experience, through which research and writing skills are learned directly through immersion in clinical studies overseen by a team of seasoned mentors. Such an experience is not offered in many doctoral degree programs, particularly online study formats.

Students in entry-level clinical doctoral programs face the same hurdles. The high cost of tuition will be an impediment to continued higher education after the entry-level clinical degree is earned. Postdoctoral positions and the continued delay of income they require will be cost prohibitive. Yet the same criteria for success will exist for health care educators in academia: scholarship through grant submission, research, and journal publication. How will health care professions answer this call? How will individual educators advance their academic careers?

This book will help educators and novice researchers better understand the skills needed for journal publication—perhaps the most essential skill for a successful academic career. The book provides specific guidelines, based on the most commonly accepted reporting standards, for the preparation and writing of general research studies, intervention effectiveness studies, instrument development and testing studies, and case reports. A section is devoted to helping authors understand the rules governing the reporting of statistical data in text and tables. Separate sections help authors understand the manuscript preparation and submission process, the revision process, and the etiquette guiding communication with editors and reviewers. Guidelines for the preparation of scholarly discussion papers and editorials are provided.

Additionally, one section aims to help doctoral students and newly minted faculty turn academic work (e.g., dissertations and theses) into publishable journal articles. In this section I also provide suggestions to help clinicians turn clinical data into research databases that could serve as the foundation for pilot studies. Lastly, I provide information to help authors better understand the ethical considerations of publication including plagiarism, dual submissions, inappropriate authorship, copyright, and conflict of interest.

The book is based on my work as an editor and author. As a former editor I was able to identify the most commonly made errors in manuscript writing and research reporting. I have compiled this knowledge in an easy-to-use-format to help authors avoid commonly made mistakes and instead develop thorough and detailed manuscripts in accordance with reporting standards accepted by the health care and scientific communities. Understanding the knowledge in this book will better help individual academicians succeed in journal publication and advance their academic careers. Such individual advancement will in turn promote health care professions as producers of respected and valued bodies of scholarship that benefit society's welfare.

REFERENCE

U.S. Department of Health and Human Services. (2015). U.S. Food and Drug Administration: Protecting and promoting your health. Retrieved from http://www.fda.gov/default.htm

2

Writing Resources—Mentors, Writing Partners, and Self-Discipline

Writing is an integral part of becoming a scholar, researcher, and academician. Our success in these roles is measured by our ability to produce published journal articles, books, research reports, grant proposals, and educational materials. While a command of English composition is prerequisite, academic authors must understand the differing style guidelines, formats, and objectives of various written materials—books, published research studies, published discussion papers, and grant applications. Each of these forms of written material requires different writing skill sets.

Sometimes academic authors can learn desired written skill sets by reading examples. Reading the articles published in professional journals can help authors better understand the formats and writing style required by specific journals. Colleagues may be willing to share accepted grant proposals to help new faculty better understand the grant writing process. Reading examples is critical, but the practice of writing multiple drafts, obtaining feedback, and making revisions is essential to learning academic writing skills. All new faculty and researchers must go through this process of drafting, obtaining feedback, and revising to become good academic writers. The process of requesting and using feedback to revise drafts of papers continues throughout an entire academic career. The best academic writers commonly seek feedback from colleagues on drafts of written materials. Feedback is commonly provided in any type of peer-reviewed submission process. For example, after authors submit a manuscript to a journal, editors and reviewers provide written feedback that the authors use to strengthen the manuscript. Novice academic authors must engage in the process of drafting, seeking feedback, and revising to gain writing expertise. To engage in this learning process, new academic authors must continuously write and become emotionally neutral in response to feedback and critique.

Gutman, S. A. *Journal Article Writing and Publication: Your Guide to Mastering Clinical Health Care Reporting Standards* (pp. 5-7). © 2017 Taylor & Francis Group.

MENTORSHIP

The most important resource when learning academic writing is having one or more seasoned academic mentors who can provide feedback on multiple drafts until the paper is published. Because academicians' workloads are often intense and they may not have time to mentor new faculty, it is sometimes beneficial for new faculty to offer paper co-authorship to secure mentorship. New faculty and researchers can also form writing support groups in which they share their writing and receive constructive critique. Participating in writing support groups can feel less intimidating than requesting feedback from a seasoned academic; however, the critique offered may not be as valuable because the group members have less experience in academic writing. Engaging in mentorship with a seasoned academic writer and participating in a writing support group are both highly recommended to help novice academic writers gain expertise.

PERSONAL COMMITMENT

While seasoned academic mentors and writing support groups are essential in the learning process, neither can enhance writing skills if authors do not make the commitment to write. To become a proficient academic writer—to become skilled and successful in journal publication, book publication, and grant submission—authors must engage in writing continuously. In other words, authors must devote a minimum of 3 hours per week to writing in one uninterrupted block of time. Attempting to write in smaller time periods will be unfruitful, because authors commonly need approximately 20 minutes to regain mental focus for a specific writing piece and begin writing where they last left off. Multitasking and writing are incompatible; authors must create a writing environment in which they are free from distractions such as cell phones, students, colleagues, clients, family, and email. Creating a distraction-free writing environment and committing to a minimum 3-hour writing period per week require time management and self-discipline. A writing time period of 3 or more hours should be scheduled into the work week along with all other work-related commitments. Honoring this scheduled time and adhering to this weekly schedule must become as sacrosanct as a covenant. To be a successful academic author, academicians must make a contract with themselves to devote time needed to write.

The more authors adhere to a weekly writing schedule, the easier it becomes to sit down at a computer, free oneself from daily distractions, and regain the flow of writing. Each time that authors reschedule their weekly writing time period or make excuses to forgo a writing session, the more difficult it becomes to regain writing flow. Soon writing projects become abandoned and the thought of writing becomes a distasteful chore that is consistently avoided.

DECREASING WRITING ANXIETY

One way that authors can prevent writing anxiety and avoidance is to outline all writing projects at the beginning and create a map or set of instructions that can be followed at each writing session. At the end of each writing session authors should make notes to themselves about how to restart writing and identify the next writing steps. The day or evening prior to their next scheduled writing session, authors should read their previous notes to direct their mental focus back to the writing project. Sleeping with those notes and directions in mind and then embarking upon writing the next day will help authors ease back into their writing.

Sometimes having a writing partner effectively helps authors commit to a weekly writing schedule and set and meet deadlines. A writing partner can be a colleague who may also be new to academia and who is similarly embarking on his or her own writing career. Writing partners can schedule appointments together to write at the library (or another quiet environment), and they can act as coaches to make sure each author is setting and adhering to deadlines.

Authors must also depersonalize feedback and recognize that it pertains to a set of sentences on a page rather than to themselves. It is also beneficial to recognize that articles are published in a polished form after multiple drafts, revisions, and professional editing. Authors must remember that first drafts, even those written by seasoned writers, often read very differently from final papers ready for publication. The more comfortable we become sharing our preliminary drafts with others, the more feedback we will receive that can ultimately help us reach publication readiness. The more we write, the less anxiety writing will cause us.

CHECKLIST FOR GATHERING AND USING WRITING RESOURCES

- Read the professional literature consistently to gain an understanding of the writing styles and formats that are used in the journals in which you wish to publish.

- Understand that writing a paper involves the development of multiple drafts, seeking feedback for each draft, and making several sets of revisions. This is a lengthy process, and one writing project can require weeks or months for completion.

- Seek a mentor who is a seasoned academic writer with a strong publication history and who can provide feedback on drafts of your written material. Cowriting with mentors and offering coauthorship on papers is a constructive solution that benefits both the learner and mentor.

- Participate in a writing support group with academic colleagues who are similarly seeking to develop writing skills in a supportive environment.

- Commit to a weekly writing schedule of 3-hour or greater blocks. Schedule this writing period into your workweek and adhere to it.

- Avoid multitasking during your 3-hour weekly writing session. Write in a nondistracting environment free of cell phones, email, and interruptions.

- Outline all writing projects before beginning to write. At the end of each writing session, make notes or a set of directions that will help you to restart writing at your next scheduled session.

- The day or night before each scheduled writing session, review your notes so that your mind begins to regain focus on the project while you sleep. Begin writing again the next day.

- If you have difficulty with self-discipline and avoid writing, seek a writing partner who is similarly a new academician with the objective of a writing career. Schedule writing sessions together and help each other set and adhere to writing deadlines.

- Depersonalize feedback and become comfortable receiving critique on written drafts. Recognize that preliminary drafts read very differently from final, publication-ready papers that have gone through multiple drafts, revisions, and professional editing.

3

Manuscript Structure and Content for General Research Studies

This section reviews in depth the basic content and structure of a research paper (*general research studies* refers to basic research and nonexperimental designs such as descriptive, qualitative, correlational, survey, longitudinal, cross-sectional, etc.). A primary concern for publishers is the cost of publication space. Even online publication has costs associated with copyediting and journal website maintenance. General manuscript length requirements are usually 5,000 words including references; however, it is critical to check the page and word count lengths in the author guidelines of the specific journal to which you intend to submit and adhere to those requirements. Not adhering to journal page length and word count will often result in returned manuscripts.

Research manuscripts for scientific, health, and social science journals should be written concisely and use the least amount of words to convey clear, in-depth meaning. There is a specific formula for writing research manuscripts that most editors and reviewers seek. Writing your research manuscript in accordance with this formatting structure will ensure that you have addressed the elements critical to clearly and transparently describe your study and reporting results. If a journal's author guidelines diverge from the following formatting structure, authors should use the structure recommended by the journal. If no structure is provided in the journal's author guidelines, use the following structure (whose heading levels are based on the *Publication Manual of the American Psychological Association*, 6th ed. [American Psychological Association, 2010]). The following headings are provided for a masked manuscript, or one in which the authors' identifying information and affiliated institutions are removed.

Gutman, S. A. *Journal Article Writing and Publication:*
Your Guide to Mastering Clinical Health Care Reporting Standards
(pp. 9-20). © 2017 Taylor & Francis Group.

MANUSCRIPT HEADINGS FOR GENERAL RESEARCH STUDIES

Title

(Begin the manuscript with a title on a separate title page. The title should be centered and typed in uppercase and lowercase letters.)

Abstract

(The Abstract should be placed on the page directly following the title page. The word *Abstract* should be capitalized and centered.)

Introduction

(The Introduction begins on the page directly following the abstract. The heading *Introduction* is not typed in the manuscript because the beginning of the manuscript text alerts the reader that the Introduction has begun.)

Method

(The Method section is positioned directly after the Introduction. The heading *Method* is centered and bolded.)

Research Design

(Research Design is the first subheading in the Method section. It is bolded and flush left.)

Participants

(Participants is the second subheading in the Method section. It is bolded and flush left.)

Instruments

(Instruments is commonly the third subheading in the Method section. It is bolded and flush left.)

Procedures

(Procedures is commonly the fourth subheading in the Method section. It is bolded and flush left.)

Data Collection

(Data Collection is the subheading that directly follows the Procedures section. It is bolded and flush left.)

Data Analysis

(Data Analysis is the subheading that directly follows the Data Collection section. It is bolded and flush left.)

Results

(The Results section directly follows the Data Analysis section and begins a new section of the manuscript. The heading *Results* is bolded and centered.)

Discussion

(The Discussion section directly follows the Results and begins a new section of the manuscript. The heading *Discussion* is bolded and centered.)

Limitations

(The Limitations subsection is part of the Discussion section but should be highlighted for the reader by a separate subheading within the Discussion section. The subheading *Limitations* is bolded and flush left.)

Future Research

(The Future Research subsection directly follows the Limitations subsection. This section is also part of the Discussion and should be highlighted for the reader by a separate subheading label. The subheading *Future Research* is bolded and flush left.)

Conclusion or Implications for Practice

(The Conclusion section, also labeled Implications for Practice, is often the final section of a manuscript. It is a new manuscript section directly following the Discussion section. The heading is bolded and centered.)

References

(References begin on a separate page following the conclusion. The heading is centered and not bolded.)

Tables

(Tables should be provided after the end of the references and should begin on a separate page. Each table should be presented on its own page. Tables are named and presented in accordance with the order in which they are mentioned in the text.)

Figures

(Figures should be provided after the end of the tables and begin on a separate page. Each figure should be presented on its own page. Figures are named and presented in accordance with the order in which they are mentioned in the text.)

MANUSCRIPT HEADING CONTENT FOR GENERAL RESEARCH STUDIES

There should be no repetition of content in the manuscript. The following sections and subsections should not contain overlap, which they will not if written as suggested.

Title

Titles help indexers categorize articles so that they can be easily accessed. If critical information is missing from titles, articles may never be accessed by their intended audience. The title of general research manuscripts should concisely describe the topic and identify the main variables examined. Titles should contain the following elements:

- The population addressed
- The independent variable (or topical issue addressed)
- The dependent variable (or topical issue addressed)
- The research design

Examples of good research manuscript titles include the following:

- Relationship Between Pencil Grasp and Handwriting Precision in 1st Graders With ADHD
- Factors That Facilitate and Impede Transition to Housing in the Chronically Homeless: A Phenomenological Study
- A Survey of Program Director Perceptions About Transitioning to OTD Entry-Level Programs

Abbreviations should be avoided unless commonly used and understood in the health care community.

Abstract

Unless otherwise specified by a journal's author guidelines, general research manuscripts should summarize the paper content using the subheadings (a) objectives, (b) method, (c) results, and (d) conclusions. Using these subheadings will ensure that you provide the reader with critical information needed to understand paper content and select papers from database searches. Although most abstracts are between 150 to 200 words, authors should check and adhere to the word count specifications outlined in a journal's author guidelines.

- Objectives: In one to two sentences, authors should describe the purpose of the study.
- Method: In one to two sentences, authors should provide information about participants (population, sample size, recruitment—convenience or random sampling, etc.), research design, and data collection procedures.
- Results: In one to two sentences, authors should report the primary findings along with statistical test results and p values.
- Conclusions: In one to two sentences, authors should describe the implications of their study for the population and profession.

Introduction

The Introduction should be approximately four to five double-spaced, typed pages and should present the background of the problem (as it relates to the population, the profession, and society), the need for the present study, and an analysis of the current related research to date. A brief review of the current related literature is embedded in the Introduction but is usually not separately labeled as "Literature Review." The review of related literature should be concisely summarized and highlight key studies and findings. Articles reviewed should have been published within the last 5 years. Classic studies published more than 5 years ago can be reviewed and are the exception to the 5-year rule. If literature published in the last 5 years is lacking, authors should clearly identify this insufficiency. After concisely reviewing the literature, authors should help readers understand the gaps existing in the current literature and the need for the present study.

The purpose statement is the final paragraph of the Introduction. Here, authors state the purpose of the present study, and research questions or hypotheses are clearly and explicitly stated. Research questions for a general research manuscript should contain the population, independent and dependent variables, and/or the topical issue examined.

Examples of good research questions include the following:

- What is the relationship between sensory processing disorders and food refusal in children with autism spectrum disorders?

- Do adolescents who are at risk for school failure demonstrate differences in cognitive problem-solving strategies compared to academically sound adolescents?

- What are the perceptions of five homeless adults who received occupational therapy services to transition from a shelter to supportive housing?

Definitions

In the Introduction and throughout the text, authors should define all new and unfamiliar terms for readers as soon as the term is presented. Many authors make the common mistakes of failing to define terms, unclearly defining terms, presenting terms early in the paper and defining them in later sections, or changing the definitions of terms in a paper. There is a formula for writing good definitions. Unless a term is technically defined in the health care community using precise language that could significantly alter the term's meaning if changed, definitions should not be quoted from another source. Instead, all definitions should either be created by the authors or paraphrased and cited.

Good definitions contain the following three elements (Mosey, 1996):

1. Label: The label is the term used to describe a specific concept. The label chosen should be used consistently throughout the paper and should not change.

2. Superordinate concept: The superordinate concept is the larger umbrella term or category under which the term falls.

3. Distinguishing characteristics: Distinguishing characteristics are the concepts that differentiate the term from similar concepts.

Examples of good definitions include the following:

1. Repetitive strain disorders are overuse syndromes in which the soft tissues of a joint become inflamed as a result of repeated engagement in activities that require continued movement.

    Repetitive strain disorders [label] are overuse syndromes [superordinate concept] in which the soft tissues of a joint become inflamed as a result of repeated engagement in activities that require continued movement [distinguishing characteristics].

2. Cognitive problem-solving strategies are executive functions mediated by the frontal lobe that require the ability to identify a problem, plan a strategy, execute the strategy, evaluate the strategy's effect, and modify the strategy as needed.

    Cognitive problem solving strategies [label] are executive functions mediated by the frontal lobe [superordinate concept] that require the ability to identify a problem, plan a strategy, execute the strategy, evaluate the strategy's effect, and modify the strategy as needed [distinguishing characteristics].

3. Food refusal is the rejection of specific food types based on tastes, textures, consistencies, scents, and appearances that are aversive to the child.

    Food refusal [label] is the rejection of specific food types [superordinate concept] based on tastes, textures, consistencies, scents, and appearances that are aversive to the child [distinguishing characteristics].

Quotations

In scholarly writing in the health sciences, quotations should only be used to quote a historical or legal document, a technical definition that has been accepted by the scientific community and whose meaning may significantly change if the exact wording is altered, or a specific participant response in a qualitative study. With the exception of the previous instances, quotations should not be used. Instead, paraphrase content and cite the source.

Method

The Method section provides a blueprint of your study procedures so that others can replicate your findings. Using the subheadings listed below to structure your Method section will ensure that you report critical and essential information needed by editors, reviewers, and readers to evaluate the quality of your methods and assess how adequately such methods addressed your study's research questions.

Research Design

Research Design should be the first subheading of the Method section because this information is needed by the reader to understand which study design has been used and whether it can adequately answer the research question. If the research design does not match the study question, the study will be flawed. When the specific research design is not clearly stated in its own section or is embedded within another section, editors and reviewers must search for this essential information. The research design should be clearly stated and described in several sentences. At the end of this subsection, authors should state that the study was approved (or exempted) by an institutional review board (or ethics committee). Authors should also state that adult participants or guardians provided consent (and that children provided assent).

Participants

Participants is the second subheading in the Methods section. The term *participants*, as opposed to *subjects*, is used in health care research to imply that those selected to participate in the study have willingly volunteered and are actively engaged in the research project. *Subjects* implies that those selected may or may not know that they are in a study and are manipulated by the researcher instead of actively participating in the research process. The term *participants* should be used consistently throughout the text.

In this subsection, authors should concisely describe the recruitment process and inclusion/exclusion criteria for study enrollment. The recruitment process description should specifically address how participants were selected (i.e., from convenience sampling or randomization, etc.), by whom, and from what setting. Both inclusion and exclusion criteria for participant selection should be explicitly stated.

Participant demographics, participant flow, and final sample size should not be addressed in this subsection; instead, this information should be provided in the beginning of the Results section.

Instruments

The third subheading in the Methods section is *Instruments*. All instruments used to measure outcomes or dependent variables should be cited and addressed with regard to intended purpose, population for which the instrument was designed and assessed, type of data collected (e.g., self-report, performance-based observer rating, Likert scale, open-ended questions, total score yielding ratio data, etc.), and administration length. An instrument's psychometric properties should be reported in numerical value with statistical test and p values indicated. All psychometric properties should be cited. If no psychometric properties have been established, or if the instrument was developed specifically for the present study, the authors should state this clearly in the Instruments section rather than addressing these conditions only in the Limitations subsection of the Discussion section. It is often helpful to readers to provide sample item questions in a table or figure when an instrument has been developed by the authors specifically for the present study.

Procedures

The *Procedures* subsection commonly follows the Instruments subsection. Here, authors should report the steps of the study in sufficient detail so the study can be replicated and so that editors, reviewers, and readers can evaluate it. Procedures should begin with steps that occurred once the study commenced. Recruitment and consent procedures should not be reported here; this information should be addressed in the Research Design and Participants subsections. To promote transparency, authors should report which researcher was responsible for and executed each specific procedure. Authors must clearly report whether researchers and participants were blinded to participant group assignment and study purpose because these conditions may significantly bias results.

Data Collection

The *Data Collection* subsection commonly follows the Instruments subsection. The data collection schedule should be clearly reported here—describing how, when, and by whom each set of data was collected. Training procedures for data collectors should be documented and if multiple data collectors were used, authors should report interrater reliability scores. Authors must also state whether data collectors were blinded to participant group assignment and whether they were different members of the research team than those who had other roles (such as participant recruiter and participant group allocator). All of this information must be provided so that editors, reviewers, and readers can evaluate whether compromised data collection procedures may have biased results. If any of the above procedures were not addressed in the study, such omissions should be disclosed in the Data Collection subsection rather than discussed only in the Limitations subsection.

Data Analysis

The final subsection of the Methods section is *Data Analysis*. Here, authors should describe and cite all statistical tests and qualitative methods used to analyze data. The use of nontraditional statistical procedures that are not congruent with traditional parametric and nonparametric data analysis should be justified and cited. Similarly, the use of statistical and qualitative analytic methods that are congruent with established norms but are not familiar to most readers should be described and cited. Authors should indicate which software program was used for statistical or qualitative data analysis, and for quantitative studies, at what significance level probability was set.

A concisely written Method section that provides all of the essential information previously listed should consist of approximately five double-spaced, typed pages.

Results

The Results section begins after the end of the Data Analysis subsection in the Method section and commences a new manuscript section. In the Results section, you will report your findings without interpreting them; interpretation of findings will be made in the Discussion section. The objective of the Results section is to report your findings in a concise, clear, and sufficient way so that readers can verify reported results. Although it is not customary to provide participant raw scores, authors are increasingly providing this information through online repositories. It is important to report the results in absolute numbers rather than percentages. When percentages are given, they should be accompanied by the absolute numbers from which percentages were derived.

Begin the Results section with information about participant flow and demographics. Participant flow includes information about the number of participants recruited, the number enrolled in the study, the number of participants who withdrew or whose participation was terminated by the researchers, and the final sample size. Reporting standards require that age, gender, race, ethnicity, education level, socioeconomic level, and topic-specific characteristics such as functional status be provided for all participants. Authors should describe power analyses, sample size estimations, and confidence level estimations that were calculated to ensure that the study sample size was adequate to yield reliable statistical results.

After participant flow and demographic information are provided, the remainder of the Results section should be organized in accordance with the order of research questions outlined in the purpose statement (of the Introduction). Findings should be reported for each research question. Missing data should be acknowledged and the protocol for handling missing data should be described. In a quantitative study, results should be reported using statistical test and p values. In a qualitative study, findings should be organized by themes with supporting participant quotations.

See Chapter 7, Reporting Statistical Data in Text and Tables, to understand how to correctly report statistical tests and symbols in the Results section.

A concisely written Results section that provides all of the essential information previously mentioned should consist of approximately three to four double-spaced, typed pages.

Discussion

The Discussion section follows the Results section and begins a new manuscript section. While the Results is a reporting of your findings without interpretation, the Discussion provides the opportunity to interpret your findings. Findings, however, should not be repeated from the Results section. For clarity, the Discussion section should be organized in accordance with the order of research questions addressed in the Results section. It is the author's objective to answer each research question based on study findings. Unexpected findings should be explained. Authors should discuss whether findings are novel or support previous work. It is critical that authors do not overstate the meaning of findings, but rather present interpretations neutrally and without qualifiers. Authors should clearly state that interpretations apply only to the study sample and not to the larger population. Readers should be left to make decisions regarding interpretation based on the presented data in the Results section.

Limitations

The Limitations subheading is inserted in the Discussion section after the previously mentioned information is addressed. Here, authors acknowledge the study limitations that may have biased the results, including small sample size, lack of control and randomization, compromised blinding procedures, and the use of assessments without established reliability and validity. Authors should discuss the generalizability of the sample to the larger population and address differences between the target population and the study sample.

Future Research

The Future Research subheading is inserted after the Limitations subheading. Here authors should indicate how future research can address the present study's limitations. Authors can also identify research questions that remain unanswered and suggest directions for future studies.

Because the separate subsections Limitations and Future Research are often brief, authors may combine them under one subheading, *Limitations and Future Research*.

A concisely and well-written Discussion section should be approximately five double-spaced, typed pages in length.

Conclusion or Implications for Practice

Most manuscripts end with a Conclusion section or a section labeled Implications for Practice. This section should summarize the study's primary findings and discuss their application to practice. A concisely, well-written Implications for Practice section should be approximately 250 to 300 words.

After the Implications for Practice section, the remaining manuscript sections in the order in which they should be presented are as follows:

- References
- Tables
- Figures

CHECKLIST FOR MANUSCRIPT STRUCTURE AND CONTENT OF GENERAL RESEARCH STUDIES

Title

- ☐ Include the population, independent variable, dependent variable, and research design.
- ☐ In a professional issue manuscript, include the topical issue in the title.

Abstract

- ☐ Objectives: In one to two sentences, describe the purpose of the study.
- ☐ Method: In one to two sentences, provide information about participants (population, sample size, recruitment—convenience or random sampling, etc.), research design, and data collection procedures.
- ☐ Results: In one to two sentences, report the primary findings along with statistical test results and p values.
- ☐ Conclusions: In one to two sentences, describe the implications of the study for the population and profession.

Introduction

- ☐ Present the background of the problem as it relates to the population, profession, and society.
- ☐ Present the need for the present study.
- ☐ Present an analysis of the current related literature to date.
- ☐ Help readers understand the gaps existing in the literature that warrant the need for the present study.
- ☐ Purpose statement: State the purpose of the present study.
- ☐ Provide primary and secondary research questions or hypotheses.
- ☐ Make sure that all terms are well defined as soon as they are presented in the manuscript.

Method

Research Design

- ☐ Describe the research design.
- ☐ State that institutional review board or ethics committee approval was obtained.

- State that participant consent was obtained (when children are participants, their parents/ guardians provide consent and children provide assent).

Participants

- Describe the recruitment process and the sampling methods through which participants were selected.
- State who completed recruitment and from what settings participants were recruited.
- Provide inclusion and exclusion criteria for participant selection.

Instruments

- Describe and cite all instruments used to measure outcomes. Describe intended purpose, population for which the instrument was designed and assessed, type of data collected (e.g., self-report, performance-based observer rating, Likert scale, open-ended questions, total score yielding ratio data, etc.), and administration length.
- Report and cite the reliability and validity for all instruments in numeric values with statistical tests and p values indicated.
- Indicate whether the instrument was developed for the present study and describe the development process; provide sample items in a table or figure if possible.

Procedures

- Report the steps of the study in sufficient detail so that the study can be evaluated and replicated by readers.
- Procedures should begin with steps that occurred once recruitment and consent procedures were completed.
- Report which researcher was responsible for and carried out each specific procedure.
- Report whether researchers and participants were blinded to participant group assignment and study purpose.

Data Collection

- Report the data collection schedule: describe how, when, and by whom each set of data was collected.
- Document the training procedures for data collectors; if multiple data collectors were used, report interrater reliability scores.
- State whether data collectors were blinded to participant group assignment.
- State whether data collectors were different from other members of the research team than those performing other roles (such as participant recruiter and participant group allocator).

Data Analysis

- Describe and cite all statistical tests and qualitative methods used to analyze data.
- Justify and cite the use of nontraditional statistical procedures that are not congruent with traditional parametric and nonparametric data analysis.
- Describe and cite the use of statistical and qualitative analytic methods that are congruent with established norms but are not familiar to most readers.
- Identify the software program used for statistical or qualitative analysis.
- For quantitative studies, state at what significance level probability was set.

Results

- Report all findings without interpreting them.
- Report results in absolute numbers rather than percentages; when percentages are provided, also indicate the absolute numbers from which percentages were derived.
- Begin the Results section with information about participant flow and demographics.
- Describe power analyses, sample size estimations, and confidence level estimations that were calculated to ensure that the study sample size was adequate to yield reliable statistical results.
- Organize the remainder of the Results section in accordance with the order of research questions outlined in the purpose statement (of the Introduction).
- Report findings for each research question.
- Acknowledge missing data and describe the protocol for handling it.
- Report quantitative findings in numerical values, with statistical tests and p values indicated.
- Organize and report qualitative findings by themes with supporting participant quotations.

Discussion

- Interpret all findings without repeating the results.
- Organize the Discussion section according to the order of research questions addressed in the Results section.
- Explain unexpected findings.
- Describe whether findings are novel or support previous work.
- Be sure that the interpretation of findings relates only to the study sample.

Limitations

- Acknowledge the study limitations that may have biased the results, including small sample size, lack of control and randomization, compromised blinding procedures, and the use of assessments without established reliability and validity.
- Discuss the generalizability of the sample to the larger population and address differences between the target population and the study sample.

Future Research

- Indicate how future research can address the present study's limitations.
- Identify research questions that remain unanswered and suggest directions for future studies.

Conclusion or Implications for Practice

- Summarize the study's primary findings and discuss their application to practice.

Examples of Well-Written General Research Journal Articles

Hwang, E. J., Peyton, C. G., Kim, D. K., Nakama-Sato, K. K., & Noble, A. E. (2014). Postdeployment driving stress and related occupational limitations among veterans of Operation Iraqi Freedom and Operation Enduring Freedom. *American Journal of Occupational Therapy, 68*(4), 386–394. doi:10.5014/ajot.2014.011668

Pollack, M. R., Metz, A. E., & Barabash, T. (2014). Association between dysfunctional elimination syndrome and sensory processing disorder. *American Journal of Occupational Therapy, 68*(4), 472–477. doi:10.5014/ajot.2014.011411

References

American Psychological Association. (2010). *Publication manual of the American Psychological Association* (6th ed.). Washington, DC: Author.

Mosey, A. C. (1996). *Applied scientific inquiry in the health professions: An epistemological orientation* (2nd ed.). Bethesda, MD: American Occupational Therapy Association.

4

Manuscript Structure and Content for Intervention Effectiveness Studies

The call for evidence-based practice has inspired health care researchers to generate studies evaluating the effect of clinical guidelines. To enhance the quality and transparency of articles describing the methods and results of clinical studies, health care stakeholders have called for the development of reporting standards for intervention studies. This chapter will focus specifically on intervention study reporting standards and the unique information that should be detailed in these types of manuscripts. The information presented next is based on American Psychological Association guidelines (2010) and the CONSORT Statement (Shulz, Altman, & Moher, 2010) and addresses manuscript structure for clinical research designs including randomized controlled studies, two-group designs with control (but no randomization), one-group pretest/posttest designs, and single-subject design studies (with several participants). Case reports with one participant are described in Chapter 6.

The headings of an intervention effectiveness manuscript are similar to those of a general research study as described in Chapter 3, and readers are urged to review this section. Using the following headings, and addressing the content that belongs in each, will help to ensure that you have included essential information sought by editors, reviewers, and readers.

Intervention effectiveness manuscripts should be approximately 5,000 words in length and 20 to 25 double-spaced, typed pages. Authors should adhere to the word and page count specifications for intervention effectiveness studies in a selected journal's author guidelines.

MANUSCRIPT HEADINGS FOR INTERVENTION EFFECTIVENESS STUDIES

The following heading levels are based on American Psychological Association guidelines formatting.

Gutman, S. A. *Journal Article Writing and Publication: Your Guide to Mastering Clinical Health Care Reporting Standards* (pp. 21-35).© 2017 Taylor & Francis Group.

Title

(Begin the manuscript with a title on a separate title page. The title should be centered and typed in uppercase and lowercase letters.)

Abstract

(The Abstract should be placed on the page directly following the title page. The word *Abstract* should be capitalized and centered.)

Introduction

(The Introduction begins on the page directly following the abstract. The heading *Introduction* is not typed in the manuscript because the beginning of the manuscript text alerts the reader that the Introduction has begun.)

Method

(The Method section is positioned directly after the Introduction. The heading *Method* is centered and bolded.)

Research Design

(*Research Design* is the first subheading in the Method section. It is bolded and flush left.)

Participants

(*Participants* is the second subheading in the Method section. It is bolded and flush left.)

Instruments

(*Instruments* is the third subheading in the Method section. It is bolded and flush left.)

Intervention

(*Intervention* is the fourth subheading in the Method sections. It is bolded and flush left.)

Intervention description.

(*Intervention description* is the first subheading of the Intervention subsection. It is indented, bolded, and ends with a period. Only the first letter of the first word is capitalized. The manuscript text begins directly after the period.)

Interveners.

(*Interveners*, or *Interventionists*, is the second subheading of the Intervention subsection. It is indented, bolded, capitalized, and ends with a period. The manuscript text begins directly after the period.)

Intervention fidelity.

(*Intervention fidelity* is the third subheading of the Intervention subsection. It is indented, bolded, and ends with a period. Only the first letter of the first word is capitalized. The manuscript text begins directly after the period.)

Data Collection

(*Data Collection* is the subheading that directly follows Intervention fidelity. It is bolded and flush left.)

Data Analysis

(*Data Analysis* is the subheading that directly follows Data Collection. It is bolded and flush left.)

Results

(The Results section directly follows Data Analysis and begins a new section of the paper. The heading *Results* is bolded and centered.)

Discussion

(The Discussion section directly follows the Results and begins a new section of the paper. The heading *Discussion* is bolded and centered.)

Limitations

(The Limitations subsection is part of the Discussion section but should be highlighted for the reader by a separate subheading within the Discussion section. The subheading *Limitations* is bolded and flush left.)

Future Research

(The Future Research subsection directly follows the Limitations subsection. This section is also part of the Discussion section and should be highlighted for the reader by a separate subheading label. The subheading *Future Research* is bolded and flush left.)

Conclusion or Implications for Practice

(The Conclusion section, also labeled Implications for Practice, is often the final section of a manuscript. It is a new manuscript section directly following the Discussion section. The heading is bolded and centered.)

References

(References begin on a separate page following the Conclusion. The heading is centered and not bolded.)

Tables

(Tables should be provided after the end of the references and begin on a separate page. Each table should be presented on its own page. Tables are named and presented in accordance with the order in which they are mentioned in the text.)

Figures

(Figures should be provided after the end of the tables and begin on a separate page. Each figure should be presented on its own page. Figures are named and presented in accordance with the order in which they are mentioned in the text.)

MANUSCRIPT HEADING CONTENT FOR INTERVENTION EFFECTIVENESS STUDIES

There should be no repetition of content in the manuscript. The sections and subsections that follow next should not contain overlap and will not if written as suggested.

Title

The title of an intervention study should contain four essential elements to help index-ers categorize the article and assist readers to clearly identify the intervention and population addressed.

1. Intervention (independent variable)

2. Targeted population

3. Outcome measures (dependent variable)

4. Research design

The acronym PICO is also used to help authors develop good titles:

- P = population

- I = intervention

- C = control or comparison (research design)

- O = outcome measures

Examples of good research titles include the following:

- Effect of a Sensory-Based Social Skill Program for Adolescents With Autism Spectrum Disorder: A Multiple-Baseline, Single-Subject Design

- Effect of a Self-Regulation Intervention for Children With ADHD: A One-Group Pretest/ Posttest Design

- Effect of an Educational Community Group for Caregivers of Adult Family Members With Dementia: A Two-Group Controlled Pretest/Posttest Design

- A Comparison of Neurodevelopmental Therapy vs Modified Constraint-Induced Therapy for Adults With Stroke: A Randomized Controlled Trial

Abbreviations in the title should be avoided unless commonly used and understood in the health care community.

Abstract

Similar to a general research manuscript, the abstract of an intervention effec-tiveness manuscript is best organized by the use of the following subheadings: (a) objectives, (b) method, (c) results, and (d) conclusions. The content of each subheading, however, differs from that of a general research manuscript with regard to intervention study details. Addressing the specific content of each subheading, as recommended next, will ensure that you provide edi-tors, reviewers, and readers with critical information needed to understand the intervention, tar-geted population, and research design. Because readers select papers primarily based on abstracts, the provision of this essential information is critical for transparent intervention effectiveness reporting.

- Objectives: In one to two sentences, authors should describe the purpose of the study.

- Method: In one to two sentences, authors should provide information about participants (pop-ulation, sample size, recruitment strategy—convenience, random sampling, etc.), research design, intervention (for treatment and control groups), length of intervention, follow-up points, and outcome measures.

- Results: In one to two sentences, authors should report the primary findings along with sta-tistical test results, p values, and effect sizes.

- Conclusions: In one to two sentences, authors should (a) describe the implications of their study for the population and profession and (b) address how the findings can be used to inform best practice.

Authors should check a specific journal's author guidelines to determine word count specifications and preferred abstract headings.

Introduction

The Introduction of an intervention effectiveness manuscript is similar to that of a general research manuscript with regard to length (four to five double-spaced, typed pages) and the need to address the background of the problem as it relates to the population, profession, and society. Because the manuscript addresses the effectiveness of a clinical practice method, however, the Introduction should focus on the intervention as it has been used with the targeted population. When reviewing the literature for readers, authors should describe the intervention's theoretical basis and/or the results of previous effectiveness studies (with the target population). Authors should identify existing knowledge gaps regarding the intervention and clearly state how the present study will contribute to the profession's best practice. The 5-year rule applies to intervention effectiveness studies—articles reviewed in the Introduction should have been published within the last 5 years; however, classic studies or theoretical papers that were published more than 5 years ago are the exception to this rule. Because many health care professions are in their early evolution in the building of evidence, intervention studies published within the last 5 years may be lacking or insufficient to make best practice decisions. When this is the case, authors should clearly describe this deficiency in the Introduction.

The purpose statement is the final paragraph of the Introduction. Here, authors should state the purpose of the intervention effectiveness study and provide clear and precise research questions. Research questions for an intervention effectiveness manuscript should contain the population, the intervention, the research design, and the outcome measures.

Examples of good research questions include the following:

- Can a client-centered, sensory-based, nutritional diet decrease food refusal in five conveniently selected children with autism spectrum disorder (ASD) compared to five conveniently selected children with ASD who received family meals as usual?

- Can a cognitive problem-solving program for 10 randomly selected adolescents at risk for school failure decrease school drop-out rates compared to matched controls?

- Can an interactive housing skill DVD program help eight conveniently selected homeless men transition from a shelter into supportive housing and maintain housing at 6-month follow-up compared to a control group that did not participate in the program?

Definitions

All new and unfamiliar terms that are presented in the Introduction (and throughout the text) should be defined when the term first appears in the manuscript. Common mistakes include failing to define terms, unclearly defining terms, presenting terms in one section and defining them in another, and changing the definition of a term in a paper. To understand how to write a good definition, authors should see Chapter 3, p. 13.

Quotations

Quotations should not be used in health science scholarly writing with the exception of the following:

- Quoting historical or legal documents

- Quoting a technical definition that has been accepted by the scientific community and whose meaning may significantly change if the exact wording is altered

- Quoting a participant's response in a qualitative study

With the exception of the above instances, quotations should not be used. Instead, authors should paraphrase content and cite the source.

Method

Providing clear, detailed, and precise methods is critical for (a) editors, reviewers, and readers to evaluate a study's internal and external validity; (b) researchers to replicate findings under similar conditions; and (c) practitioners to understand whether an intervention can be applied to their own clients and clinical setting. Transparency in reporting is essential to understand whether an intervention demonstrates effectiveness with a specific clinical population and whether findings can be generalized beyond the study sample. If authors do not provide the essential information to determine the above, manuscripts cannot be evaluated and are often rejected. The use of the following subheadings in the Method section, and the content belonging in each subheading, will help you to provide critical information that editors and reviewers seek.

Research Design

The Method section of intervention effectiveness manuscripts should begin with a subheading labeled *Research Design*. Detailing the design is critical for readers to understand whether the design can truly answer the research questions and address effectiveness. When authors do not describe the research design or embed it in another section, it is difficult for editors and reviewers to evaluate the study. The type of design should be explicitly labeled (e.g., randomized controlled trial, two-group pretest/posttest with control, one-group pretest/posttest, single subject design, crossover design, or factorial design). Description of the design should include the number and type of participant groups (treatment and control), whether control or randomization was used, when measurements were administered, and whether follow-up data collection measures were used. Authors should state that institutional review board (or ethics committee) approval was obtained (or exempted) and that participant/guardian consent was attained. If children served as participants, authors should indicate whether parental or guardian consent was obtained and whether children provided assent.

Participants

The Participants subsection specifically addresses recruitment procedures and inclusion and exclusion criteria. Authors should explicitly state the type of sampling method used to recruit participants (e.g., convenience or randomization), who recruited participants, and from what setting. If randomization was used, authors should specify the method through which the random sequence assignment was generated, whether the recruiter was blinded to the random assignment process, and whether the researcher who created the random assignment process was different from the researcher who enrolled and assigned participants to groups. All of these methods serve to reduce potential sampling bias. Similarly, if nonrandomized control groups or matching was used, authors should describe what method was used to assign participants to group conditions or as matched controls.

Inclusion and exclusion criteria should be clearly provided in sufficient detail so that readers can understand who was (and who was not) the targeted participant group, how similarly this group matched the larger population, and whether the targeted participant group was actually recruited and enrolled in the study. The setting(s) from which participants were recruited should be detailed; participants from varying settings may have different demographics and motives for participation that may be otherwise difficult to discern if not specified in this section. Description of facility type and geographical region should be noted.

Participant demographics, participant flow, and final sample size are part of the results and should be documented in the Results section rather than the Method section.

Instruments

Documentation of the instruments through which you measured your outcomes is essential since outcomes provide information about intervention effectiveness. Instruments should be described in detail so that readers can evaluate whether a selected instrument was appropriate to measure a specific outcome. If inappropriate instruments were used to measure specific outcomes, the findings will have no bearing on the intervention's genuine effectiveness. Instruments should be described with regard to purpose, intended population, type of data collected (e.g., self-report, performance based observer rating, Likert scale, open-ended questions, or total score yielding ratio data), and administration length. The instrument's psychometric properties relating to reliability and validity should be provided in numeric values, with statistical tests and *p* values indicated. It is insufficient to state that the instrument's reliability or validity is *high*; readers should be provided with the numeric values of statistical tests so that they can evaluate the instrument themselves. Both the instrument and the psychometric properties should be cited. If psychometric properties for an instrument have not been established, or if an instrument has been newly developed for the present intervention study, the authors should state this information in the Instruments section. Using an instrument without established psychometric properties for an intervention effectiveness study will yield findings that may not be reliable. Authors should justify their decision to use such an instrument in this section. Waiting for the Limitations subsection of the Discussion to disclose this information will appear as though this critical information has been withheld from readers.

Similarly, if authors have developed an instrument for the present intervention effectiveness study, they should at minimum describe the development process and disclose whether an attempt was made to establish face or content validity through the evaluation of an expert panel. If space permits, sample items can be illustrated in a table or figure.

Intervention

The intervention section is unique to intervention effectiveness studies and case reports and is divided into three subsections listed below.

1. *Intervention description.* Authors should describe the intervention and state if the intervention is manualized (or based on a written set of guidelines for practice and training that can be accessed by others). Key elements should be provided, addressing the number and length of sessions and the length of intervention over time, the content of each session and whether sessions were delivered individually or in a group, and whether and how the intervention was tailored for specific clients. Authors should also disclose whether clients received any type of simultaneous clinical service that could have influenced results. If a control group was used, authors should provide the above information for both treatment and control groups.

2. *Interveners.* Key information should be provided about the professionals who administered the intervention. Authors should report the type of professional and number of therapists who administered the intervention, the criteria used to select therapists, therapist experience level, the type of training received to administer the intervention, and whether therapists were blinded to participant group assignment. If a control group was used, authors should disclose whether the same therapist(s) provided intervention to the treatment and control group.

3. *Intervention fidelity.* Intervention fidelity refers to the procedures used to ensure that the intervention was administered in accordance with a written manual, particularly if more than one intervener was used. Authors should describe the procedures used to ensure intervention fidelity and document whether intervention fidelity was measured using an objective instrument. If intervention fidelity was not assessed, authors should explicitly state this here rather than wait for the Limitations section.

All of the above information is necessary for readers to replicate the study and understand whether potential bias occurred that could weaken the reliability of results. If any of the above items were not addressed in the study, it is better for authors to disclose such conditions in this section. Waiting to disclose weaknesses in the Limitations section may cause readers to think that key information regarding study design flaws has been withheld.

Data Collection

The Data Collection subsection should detail how, when, and by whom each set of data in the study was collected. Authors should describe the data collection schedule (i.e., when each set of data was collected and by whom), how data collectors were trained to collect data uniformly, whether interrater reliability was established for data collectors if more than one data collector was used, and whether data collectors were blinded to participant group assignment. It is critical to disclose whether data collectors were different from interveners or if interveners also collected data; the latter condition introduces possible bias that could influence findings regarding the genuine effectiveness of the intervention.

Data Analysis

In the Data Analysis subsection, authors should detail the statistical procedures that were used to compare pre- and postintervention measures and provide citations for all statistical methods. When statistical methods were used that are not congruent with traditional parametric and nonparametric rules of data analysis, authors should justify chosen methods and provide citation. Statistical methods that are congruent with traditional data analysis procedures but will likely be unfamiliar to readers should also be justified and cited. Authors should indicate and cite the software program used to generate statistical calculations and report the level at which statistical significance was set. If a randomized or nonrandomized controlled trial was conducted, it is important to report whether intention-to-treat analysis (ITT) was performed (Gupta, 2011). In ITT analysis, all participants enrolled in a study are included in the final data analysis regardless of whether they received treatment and completed the study. ITT analysis mirrors treatment changes and nonadherence that commonly occur in practice and factors these conditions into the analysis of intervention effectiveness. When study noncompleters are removed from final data analysis, bias is introduced in favor of treatment effectiveness. ITT reduces bias and provides a fuller understanding of intervention effectiveness.

The Method section should be approximately five double-spaced, typed pages in length.

Results

The Results section should begin with a description of participant flow including the number of participants recruited, the number enrolled, the number assigned to each group condition, the number who received follow-up measures, and the number included in the final analysis. In randomized controlled trials and two-group pretest/posttest designs with control, participant flow should be illustrated using a flow chart (Figure 4-1). Authors should indicate whether ITT analysis was performed and clearly state the (a) number of participants who withdrew (or were withdrawn by the researcher) and for what reasons, if known; (b) the number who were lost to follow-up; and (c) the number who did not adhere to intervention recommendations (and for what reasons, if known). All adverse events occurring as a result of the intervention (in both treatment and control groups) should be reported.

Authors should report participant demographics with regard to age, gender, race, ethnicity, education level, socioeconomic level, and topic-specific characteristics such as functional level and independent living status. When demographics are reported, absolute numbers should be provided. If percentages are used, the absolute numbers from which the percentages were derived should be provided. If any of the above-noted demographics were not collected, authors should disclose this.

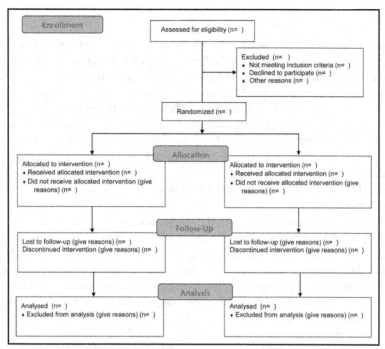

Figure 4-1. CONSORT 2010 Flow Diagram.

When reporting the sample size, authors should indicate whether a power analysis was performed to estimate the minimum sample size needed to avoid a Type II error (or an error in which the intervention is believed to be ineffective when in fact it is effective).

After reporting participant flow and demographics, authors should provide information about the equivalence of control and intervention groups (when comparison or control is used). Procedures used to establish whether control and intervention groups were statistically equivalent on baseline measures should be described. If statistically significant differences exist between the control and intervention groups at baseline, authors should detail the statistical methods used to control or remove differences.

When comparison or control groups are used, authors should report between-group outcomes first. If between-group outcome measures are not statistically significant, it is difficult to justify intervention effectiveness. A common mistake involves the minimization of statistically insignificant between-group differences while highlighting statistically significant within-group findings. In this situation, it is inappropriate to use within-group findings to justify the effectiveness of the intervention when in fact no statistically significant differences exist between the intervention group and the control or comparison.

When reporting results, the statistical test value, p value, and effect size should be reported. Effect size allows readers to evaluate whether statistically significant differences between groups (and pre- and posttests) are large enough to be clinically meaningful. Confidence intervals, which indicate the range of uncertainty for the intervention effect, should also be reported.

Authors should disclose the existence of missing data and describe the statistical methods for handling missing data. Authors should also report whether the intervention was carried out as intended and provide objective data confirming intervention fidelity, if measures were used.

See Chapter 7, Reporting Statistical Data in Text and Tables, to understand how to correctly report statistical tests and symbols in the Results section.

The Results section should be between three and four double-spaced pages in length.

Discussion

The Discussion section allows authors to interpret their findings for readers. It is critical, however, that authors do not overstate or inflate intervention effectiveness. Findings about the intervention's effectiveness should always be interpreted with caution and the acknowledgement that interpretations can only be applied to the study sample (rather than the larger population). Findings should also be discussed with regard to efficacy and effectiveness. *Efficacy* refers to the effect of an intervention under the tightly controlled conditions of a research setting. *Effectiveness* refers to the effect of an intervention under the practical, real-life conditions of a clinical setting. An intervention that demonstrates efficacy with a specific population under tightly controlled research conditions may not be as potent in a real-life clinical setting in which patient adherence and acceptance, daily time restraints, therapist skill level, and available resources can affect intervention feasibility and outcome.

The Discussion section should be organized in accordance with the order of research questions provided in the purpose statement and addressed in the Results section. Authors should attempt to answer each research question based on findings provided in the Results section. Unanticipated findings should be explained, and authors should discuss whether intervention effectiveness findings are novel or support previous studies. Because several intervention studies are required before consensus can be established regarding intervention effectiveness for a specific population, authors should refrain from suggesting that the intervention in question is effective beyond the study sample unless their research supports a body of already established evidence. If a body of research has not been established, authors should explain how their findings contribute to a growing consensus regarding best practice.

Limitations

Confounding variables that may have reduced the study's internal and external validity should be acknowledged. Factors weakening the study's internal validity—the degree to which researchers can be confident that the intervention was responsible for changes in outcome measures—should be addressed. These include lack of intervention fidelity, compromised blinding procedures of the interveners and/or data collectors, varying therapist skill level, insufficient sample size power, lack of control and/or randomization, and use of assessments having weak or no established psychometric properties. Factors weakening external validity—the degree to which researchers can be confident that the participants represent the larger population—should be detailed. These include compromised blinding procedures of the group allocator, biased recruitment and enrollment, compromised sampling methods, and the possible influence of participant incentives. A further limitation of many intervention effectiveness studies is lack of follow-up points, without which researchers cannot understand whether the intervention's effect lasted over time.

Future Research

Authors should suggest how future studies can address the present study's limitations and identify which questions regarding intervention use must still be answered. For example, is the intervention cost and time efficient? Can patients tolerate the intervention, and if not, how can it be improved? Although the intervention has been found to be effective with children, can it be used with adolescents and adults having the same diagnosis?

The Discussion section should be approximately four to five pages in length.

Conclusion or Implications for Practice

In this final section of the manuscript text, authors should summarize the major study findings and describe how these can be applied in practice.

After the Implications for Practice, the remaining manuscript sections in the order in which they should be presented are as follows:

- References
- Tables
- Figures

CHECKLIST FOR MANUSCRIPT STRUCTURE AND CONTENT OF INTERVENTION EFFECTIVENESS STUDIES

Title

☐ Include the following elements: intervention (independent variable), targeted population, outcome measures (dependent variable), research design (control, comparison)

Abstract

☐ Objectives: In one to two sentences, describe the purpose of the study.

☐ Method: In one to two sentences, provide information about participants (population, sample size, recruitment strategy—convenience, random sampling, etc.), research design, intervention (for treatment and control groups), length of intervention, follow-up points, and outcome measures.

☐ Results: In one to two sentences, report the primary findings along with statistical test results, p values, and effect sizes.

☐ Conclusions: In one to two sentences, (a) describe the implications of the study for the population and profession and (b) address how the findings can be used to inform best practice.

Introduction

☐ Describe the background of the problem as it relates to the population, profession, and society.

☐ Describe the intervention's use with the targeted population, the intervention's theoretical base, and the results of previous intervention effectiveness studies with the population.

☐ Identify existing knowledge gaps regarding the intervention and clearly state how the present study will contribute to the profession's best practice.

☐ Purpose statement: state the purpose of the intervention effectiveness study.

☐ Provide primary and secondary research questions.

☐ Make sure that all terms are well defined as soon as they are presented in the manuscript.

Method

Research Design

☐ Describe the research design (e.g., randomized controlled trial, two-group pretest/posttest with control, one-group pretest/posttest, single-subject design, crossover design, or factorial design).

- Include the number and type of participant groups (treatment and control), whether control or randomization was used, when measurements were administered, and whether follow-up data collection measures were used.

- State that institutional review board (or ethics committee) approval was obtained (or exempted) or that participant or guardian consent was attained. If children served as participants, indicate whether parental or guardian consent was obtained and whether children provided assent.

Participants

- State the type of sampling method used to recruit participants (e.g., convenience, randomization), who recruited participants, and from what setting.

- If randomization was used, specify the method through which the random sequence assignment was generated, whether the recruiter was blinded to the random assignment process, and whether the researcher who created the random assignment process was different from the researcher who enrolled and assigned participants to groups.

- If nonrandomized control groups or matching was used, describe what method was used to assign participants to group conditions or as matched controls.

- Provide inclusion and exclusion criteria in sufficient detail so that readers can understand who was (and who was not) the targeted participant group, how similarly this group matched the larger population, and whether the targeted participant group was actually recruited and enrolled in the study.

- If one or more sites were used, describe the facility types and geographical region.

Instruments

- Describe instruments with regard to purpose, intended population, type of data collected (e.g., self-report, performance-based observer rating, Likert scale, open-ended questions, total score yielding ratio data, etc.), and administration length. Cite all instruments.

- Provide and cite the instrument's psychometric properties in numeric values, with statistical tests and p values indicated.

- Justify the use of instruments with little or no established psychometric properties.

- If an instrument was developed for the present intervention effectiveness study, describe the development process and whether an attempt was made to establish face or content validity through the evaluation of an expert panel. Sample items can be illustrated in a table or figure.

Intervention

Intervention Description

- Describe the intervention and state whether the intervention is manualized (or based on a written set of guidelines for practice and training that can be accessed by others).

- Provide information about the number and length of sessions and the length of intervention over time, the content of each session and whether sessions were delivered individually or in a group, and whether and how the intervention was tailored for specific clients.

- Indicate whether clients received any type of simultaneous clinical service that could have influenced results.

- Provide all of the above information for both treatment and control groups (if controls were used).

Interveners

☐ Report the type of professional and number of therapists who administered the intervention, criteria used to select therapists, therapist experience level, type of training received to administer the intervention, and whether therapists were blinded to participant group assignment.

☐ If a control group was used, disclose whether the same therapist(s) provided intervention to the treatment and control group.

Intervention Fidelity

☐ Describe the procedures used to ensure intervention fidelity and document whether intervention fidelity was measured using an objective instrument.

☐ Clearly indicate whether intervention fidelity was not addressed.

Data Collection

☐ Describe the data collection schedule (i.e., when each set of data was collected in the study and by whom).

☐ Describe how data collectors were trained to collect data uniformly and whether interrater reliability was established for data collectors if more than one data collector was used.

☐ Describe whether data collectors were blinded to participant group assignment.

☐ Disclose whether data collectors were different from interveners.

Data Analysis

☐ Describe and cite the statistical procedures that were used to compare pre- and postintervention measures.

☐ Justify and cite the use of statistical methods that are not congruent with traditional parametric and nonparametric rules of data analysis.

☐ Cite the use of statistical methods that may be unfamiliar to readers.

☐ Indicate and cite the software program used to generate statistical calculations and report the level at which statistical significance was set.

☐ If a randomized or nonrandomized controlled trial was conducted, report whether intention-to-treat analysis was performed.

Results

☐ Begin the Results section with a description of participant flow including the number of participants recruited, the number enrolled, the number assigned to each group condition, the number who received follow-up measures, and the number included in the final analysis.

☐ In randomized controlled trials and two-group pretest/posttest designs with control, illustrate participant flow with a flow chart.

☐ Indicate whether ITT analysis was performed and clearly state the (a) number of participants who withdrew (or were withdrawn by the researcher) and for what reasons, if known; (b) the number who were lost to follow-up; and (c) the number who did not adhere to intervention recommendations (and for what reasons, if known).

☐ Report all adverse events occurring as a result of the intervention (in both treatment and control groups).

☐ Report participant demographics with regard to age, gender, race, ethnicity, education level, socioeconomic level, and topic-specific characteristics such as functional level and independent living status.

- Describe power analyses, sample size estimations, and confidence level estimations that were calculated to ensure that the study sample size was adequate to yield reliable statistical results.
- Provide information about the equivalence of control and intervention groups (when comparison or control is used).
- When reporting results, the statistical test value, p value, and effect size should be reported.
- Acknowledge the existence of missing data and describe the statistical methods for handling missing data.
- Report whether the intervention was carried out as intended and provide objective data confirming intervention fidelity.

Discussion

- Interpret all findings without repeating the results.
- Organize the Discussion section according to the order of research questions addressed in the Results section.
- Explain unexpected findings.
- Describe whether findings are novel or support previous work.
- Be sure that the interpretation of findings relates only to the study sample.

Limitations

- Acknowledge factors weakening internal validity.
  - Lack of intervention fidelity, compromised blinding procedures of the interveners and/or data collectors, varying therapist skill level, insufficient sample size power, lack of control and/or randomization, and use of assessments having weak or no established psychometric properties.
- Acknowledge factors weakening external validity.
  - Compromised blinding procedures of the group allocator, biased recruitment and enrollment, compromised sampling methods, and the possible influence of participant incentives.

Future Research

- Suggest how future studies can address the present study's limitations and identify which questions regarding intervention use must still be answered.

Conclusion or Implications for Practice

- Summarize the major study findings and describe how these can be applied in practice.

EXAMPLES OF WELL-WRITTEN INTERVENTION EFFECTIVENESS JOURNAL ARTICLES

Case-Smith, J., DeLuca, S. C., Stevenson, R., & Ramey, S. L. (2012). Multicenter randomized controlled trial of pediatric constraint-induced movement therapy: 6-month follow-up. *American Journal of Occupational Therapy, 66*(1), 15–23. doi:10.5014/ajot.2012.002386

Gutman, S. A., Raphael-Greenfield, E. I., & Rao, A. K. (2012). Effect of a motor-based role-play intervention on the social behaviors of adolescents with high-functioning autism: Multiple-baseline single-subject design. *American Journal of Occupational Therapy, 66,* 529–537. doi:10.5014/ajot.2012.003756

REFERENCES

American Psychological Association. (2010). *Publication manual of the American Psychological Association* (6th ed.). Washington, DC: Author.

Gupta, S. K. (2011). Intention-to-treat concept: A review. *Perspectives in Clinical Research, 2*(3), 109–112. doi:10.4103/2229-3485.83221

Schulz, K. F., Altman, D. G., & Moher, D., for the CONSORT Group. (2010). CONSORT 2010 Statement: Updated guidelines for reporting parallel group randomized trials. *British Medical Journal, 340,* c332. doi:10.1136/bmj.c332

5

Manuscript Structure and Content for Instrument Development and Testing Studies

Instrument development and testing studies hold great significance for a health profession's advancement because intervention effectiveness cannot be demonstrated without reliable and valid assessments. Without studies that establish the psychometric properties of instruments, evidence-based research and practice cannot occur. It is critical that health professions develop reliable and valid instruments that measure the services they render. For example, although occupational therapists help people with disabilities to enhance functional performance in daily occupations and community participation, the profession is in the beginning stages of developing assessments that measure functional daily activity in the home and community. Such instruments are considered to be ecologically valid and more accurately address the outcomes of occupational therapy practice. When occupational therapists use assessments developed by other professionals that do not address function in the context of real-life activities, reliable information cannot be discerned about the effectiveness of occupational therapy services.

Similar to intervention effectiveness manuscripts, there is a uniform way to report the findings of instrument development and testing studies that promotes transparency and allows readers to assess whether the standards for good methodological quality have been met. This section will focus on the unique content and structure of instrument development and testing study manuscripts and is based on the consensus-based standards for the selection of health status measurement instruments (COSMIN) (Mokkink et al., 2010).

The length of instrument development and testing studies varies depending on the number of psychometric properties addressed in the study; however, authors should aim for a length between 4,000 and 5,000 words including references.

Gutman, S. A. *Journal Article Writing and Publication: Your Guide to Mastering Clinical Health Care Reporting Standards* (pp. 37-50). © 2017 Taylor & Francis Group.

MANUSCRIPT HEADINGS FOR INSTRUMENT DEVELOPMENT AND TESTING STUDIES

The following heading levels are based on American Psychological Association (2010) formatting.

Title

(Begin the manuscript with a title on a separate title page. The title should be centered and typed in uppercase and lowercase letters.)

Abstract

(The Abstract should be placed on the page directly following the title page. The word *Abstract* should be capitalized and centered.)

Introduction

(The Introduction begins on the page directly following the abstract. The heading *Introduction* is not typed in the manuscript because the beginning of the manuscript text alerts the reader that the Introduction has begun.)

Method

(The Method section is positioned directly after the Introduction. The heading *Method* is bolded and centered.)

Research Design

(*Research Design* is the first subheading in the Method section. It is bolded and flush left.)

Participants

(*Participants* is the second subheading in the Method section. It is bolded and flush left.)

Instruments

(*Instruments* is the third subheading in the Method section. It is bolded and flush left.)

Procedures

(*Procedures* is the fourth subheading in the Method section. It is bolded and flush left.)

Data Collection

(*Data Collection* is the subheading that directly follows Procedures. It is bolded and flush left.)

Data Analysis

(*Data Analysis* is the subheading that directly follows Data Collection. It is bolded and flush left.)

Results

(The Results section directly follows Data Analysis and begins a new section of the paper. The heading *Results* is bolded and centered.)

Discussion

(The Discussion section directly follows the Results and begins a new section of the paper. The heading *Discussion* is bolded and centered.)

Limitations

(The Limitations subsection is part of the Discussion section but should be highlighted for the reader by a separate subheading within the Discussion section. The subheading *Limitations* is bolded and flush left.)

Future Research

(The Future Research subsection directly follows the Limitations subsection. It is also part of the Discussion section and should be highlighted for the reader by a separate subheading. The subheading *Future Research* is bolded and flush left.)

Conclusion or Implications for Practice

(The Conclusion section, also labeled Implications for Practice, is often the final section of a manuscript. It is a new manuscript section directly following the Discussion section. The heading is bolded and centered.)

References

(References begin on a separate page following the Conclusion. The heading is centered and not bolded.)

Tables

(Tables should be provided after the end of the references and begin on a separate page. Each table should be presented on its own page. Tables are named and presented in accordance with the order in which they are mentioned in the text.)

Figures

(Figures should be provided after the end of the tables and begin on a separate page. Each figure should be presented on its own page. Figures are named and presented in accordance with the order in which they are mentioned in the text.)

MANUSCRIPT HEADING CONTENT FOR INSTRUMENT DEVELOPMENT AND TESTING STUDIES

There should be no repetition of content in the manuscript. The sections and subsections mentioned next should not contain overlap and will not if written as suggested.

Title

Providing essential elements in the title of an instrument development and testing study will ensure that the study reaches researchers and practitioners interested in the instrument's use.

Titles of instrument studies should contain the following three elements:

1. The population
2. The instrument name or the construct measured
3. The psychometric properties addressed

The following are examples of good titles for instrument development and testing studies:

- Interrater Reliability of the Home Assessment Scale for Elderly With Low Vision
- Content Validity of the Mild Brain Injury Assessment for Children in the Classroom
- Convergent Validity Between Driving Simulators and On-Road Assessments in Adults With Parkinson's Disease

Abbreviations should be avoided unless commonly used and understood in the health care community.

Abstract

Authors should check a specific journal's author guidelines to determine the formatting requirements for abstracts. Unless specified otherwise, the abstract for instrument development and testing manuscripts should be organized by the following subheadings: (a) objectives, (b) method, (c) results, and (d) conclusions. Using these subheadings—and the content required in each subheading—will ensure that you provide readers with critical information about the instrument, the construct measured, the targeted population, and the quality of the methodology and findings. Most abstracts are between 150 and 200 words; however, authors should check and adhere to the word count specifications outlined in a journal's author guidelines.

- Objectives: In one to two sentences, authors should describe the purpose of the study, which will address the development or further refinement of an instrument and/or the assessment of its psychometric properties.

- Method: In one to two sentences, authors should provide information about the research design, study timeline, participants (population, sample size), and data collection procedures.

- Results: In one to two sentences, authors should report the primary findings along with statistical test results as calculated using either classical test theory (CTT) or item response theory (IRT).

- Conclusions: In one to two sentences, authors should describe the implications of their findings for the instrument's use with the targeted population.

Introduction

The Introduction of an instrument study should describe the background of the problem as it relates to the population, profession, and society (i.e., the need for an instrument that measures a specific construct with a targeted population to enhance evaluation and practice). Information about the incidence of the population for which the instrument has been targeted should be provided with recent citations. The impact of the diagnosis or clinical problem on functional community participation should be discussed so that readers understand the significance of the clinical problem as it relates to the larger society. The construct measured by the instrument should be defined; all novel or unfamiliar terms should also be defined as soon as they are presented in the manuscript (see information about writing good definitions in Chapter 3, p. 13).

As mentioned earlier, a critical need for the development of many occupational therapy assessments relates to the lack of established instruments having ecological validity, or the ability to measure a patient's functional performance in real-life everyday activities. The need for most instrument studies will address this problem or one of the following situations:

- The instrument has been recently developed and requires the establishment of psychometric properties.
- The psychometric properties of an instrument have been established using CTT but could be strengthened using IRT.
- The instrument has been revised, and psychometric properties must be established for the revision (e.g., a short version of an instrument has been newly developed based on the original long version).
- The instrument was developed in one language, and psychometric properties were established for that version. The instrument has now been translated into another language, and psychometric properties must be established for the translated version.

Authors should discuss the literature examining the assessment of the construct with the targeted population through the use of other instruments. The need for the newly developed or revised instrument in the present study should be made clear against the context of previous measures or lack thereof. Authors should briefly describe the instrument (a detailed description of the instrument will be made in the Method section), and for newly developed instruments, the theoretical base should be provided.

The purpose statement is positioned in the final paragraph of the Introduction section. Here authors should clearly and concisely detail the need to establish specific psychometric properties of an instrument to help researchers and practitioners understand how well the assessment can be used to evaluate patient or participant performance. Either precise research questions or hypotheses should be provided. Research questions should include the targeted population, the instrument name (or names if convergent or criterion validity is examined), and the psychometric property or properties examined. Hypotheses should be formulated a priori (before data collection) and include the direction and magnitude of expectations.

The following are examples of good research questions for instrument development and testing studies:

- Is the Sensory Profile reliable for use with children with mental health diagnoses?
- What is the construct and content validity of the Evaluation of Social Skills Scale for Children with Autism?
- What is the convergent validity of two PTSD scales for veterans: Impact of Events Scale and Mississippi Scale for Combat-Related PTSD?

Quotations

As stated in Chapters 3 and 4, quotations should only be used in scholarly writing when quoting a historical source or legal document; presenting a specific definition accepted by the scientific community, whose meaning would change if the exact wording were altered; and verbatim responses from patients or clients. With the exception of these instances, quotations should be avoided in health care writing. Authors should instead paraphrase and cite the original source.

A concisely and well-written Introduction section should be approximately three to four double-spaced, typed pages in length.

Method

Research Design

Authors should begin the Method section with the subheading *Research Design*. Here, the specific design should be stated and described beyond simply noting that the study involved the assessment of psychometric properties. The specific types of reliability and/or validity assessed should be stated and defined, and authors should indicate whether the design is based on CTT or IRT. Authors must also indicate whether the design involves retrospective (i.e., data that have been collected as part of practice before the commencement of the study) or prospective (i.e., data that are collected as part of the present study) data collection. The Research Design section should end with a statement that the research study received institutional review board or ethics committee approval (or exemption) and that participants provided consent (for a prospective study).

Participants

The Participants subsection in the Method section details how and from where the participants were selected, the type of sampling method used, and inclusion and exclusion criteria. The Participants section allows readers to understand the characteristics of the targeted population rather than the actual sample that was enrolled and completed the study. In an instrument study, researchers must select a sample that adequately reflects the target population; otherwise findings about instrument reliability and validity derived from a sample that does not match the intended population will be meaningless. For example, if researchers design an instrument for adults with mental health concerns but attempt to establish instrument reliability with healthy college students, reliability data derived from the sample of healthy college students will not yield genuine information about the instrument's reliability with adults with mental illness. The inclusion and exclusion criteria should be explicitly stated and in a retrospective study should detail how patient medical records were selected. Sampling methods and the settings from which participants were selected should be documented; such information is important for editors, reviewers, and readers to assess potential sampling bias and incongruence between the larger population and sample.

Instruments

Although the instrument assessed in the study was briefly introduced in the Introduction, authors must provide specific details about it in this section. The following should be documented: the instrument purpose, intended population, type of data collected (e.g., self-report, performance based observer rating, Likert scale, open-ended questions, or total score yielding ratio data), and administration length. The setting in which the instrument was intended to be administered should be described, particularly because performance-based instruments should be used in real-life activities within the community to obtain genuine information about patient daily function. If any previous psychometric properties regarding reliability, validity, and responsiveness were established, these should be noted with citations. When convergent and criterion validity are assessed, the comparison instrument should be described in detail with regard to the above information.

Procedures

The Procedures subsection should document the process of instrument development, revision, or translation (if applicable); the procedures through which reliability, validity, and/or responsiveness were assessed; the study timeline and sequence of events; and the setting in which instrument administration occurred.

Content Validity

In a content validity study authors should indicate whether an assessment was performed to determine the following:

- Whether all test items refer to relevant aspects of the construct and collectively reflect the construct
- Whether all items are relevant for the study population with regard to age, gender, disease characteristics, geographical region/country, setting
- Whether a table of specifications was used to determine the number, range, and content of instrument items
- Whether a panel of content experts was used to assess content validity

Convergent and Criterion Validity

- In a convergent or criterion validity study authors should document the steps used to ensure that the comparison instrument was a reasonable gold standard or best available instrument for comparison.

- In such studies evaluators should be blinded to the other measures to minimize the risk of expectation and limit biased ratings.

Reliability

For assessment of reliability including interrater, intrarater, and test-retest, authors should report the following:

- Whether at least two measurements were available for comparison

- Whether the instrument administrations were independent of each other—the first administration did not influence the second

- The time interval between instrument administrations (2 weeks is customary for most reliability studies and is considered long enough to reduce the risk of item recall but short enough to limit the possibility that the patient did not maintain stability on the construct being measured)

- Whether patients were stable on the construct measured over the 2-week period of instrument administration

- Whether conditions were the same for both instrument administrations (i.e., setting, type of instructions provided)

- For interrater reliability, whether raters were blinded to each other's scores to reduce bias

For internal consistency—the degree to which all instrument items reflect the same underlying construct—authors should report whether scale unidimensionality was checked. Scale unidimensionality refers to the degree to which a scale measures one construct.

Translation Studies

When an instrument has been translated into another language, authors should indicate the following:

- The expertise level of the translators with regard to language translation, knowledge of the diagnosis, and knowledge of the construct measured by the instrument

- Whether the translators worked independently of each other

- Whether back and forward translations were performed

- How differences between the original and translated instrument versions were resolved

- Whether the translation was reviewed by a panel of experts

- Whether the translated instrument was pretested to check for possible problems in interpretation, cultural relevance, and understandability

Data Collection

In the Data Collection subsection authors should describe the sequence of the data collection schedule and how and by whom data were collected. Data collectors should be described in terms of type of professional, expertise level, and training in data collection procedures. Such elements are critical for editors, reviewers, and readers to evaluate whether data collection may have been biased by differences among data collector training and experience. Blinding is a crucial element used to reduce the risk that data collectors were influenced by each other, separate test administrations, and participant scores.

- In convergent and criterion validity studies, authors should indicate whether data collectors were blinded to the other instrument and participant scores to reduce expectation bias.

- In interrater reliability studies, authors should indicate whether data collectors were blinded to each other's scores.

Data Analysis

In instrument development and testing studies, authors must indicate whether data analysis was based on CTT or IRT, as this will determine the appropriateness of the selected statistical models and tests. When using CTT, authors should describe and cite all statistical test methods. The use of nontraditional statistical procedures that are incongruent with traditional parametric and nonparametric data analysis should be justified and cited. The use of statistical tests that may be congruent with traditional parametric and nonparametric data analysis but are likely unfamiliar to readers should also be justified and cited. Authors should identify and cite the software program used to generate statistical analysis and indicate at what significance level probability was set.

When using IRT, authors should describe the model (e.g., one-parameter logistic model, OPLM; partial credit model, PCM; graded response model, GRM) and the software program (e.g., RUMM2020, WINSTEPS, OPLM, MULTILOG, PARSCALE, BILOG, NLMIXED). Authors should also report the method of estimation used (e.g., conditional maximum likelihood, CML; marginal maximum likelihood, MML) and identify the assumptions for estimating parameters of the IRT model (unidimensionality; local independence; and item fit, differential item functioning or DIF).

A concisely and well-written Method section should be approximately four to five double-spaced, typed pages in length.

Results

Although most instrument development and testing studies in education and social science do not report information about participant flow, information about the number of participants who withdrew (or were withdrawn by the researcher) because they could not tolerate test conditions is critical in the reporting of health care instruments. The Results section should begin with information about participant flow (particularly the number enrolled, the number withdrawn due to intolerance of testing conditions and why, and the final sample size) and participant demographics. Participant demographics should be reported in terms of age, gender, race, ethnicity, education level, socioeconomic level, and topic-specific characteristics such as functional status. Demographics should be reported in absolute numbers; if percentages are provided, the absolute number from which the percentage was derived should also be reported. The reporting of participant demographics is critical for readers to evaluate whether your sample matched the larger population; if it did not, psychometric properties reported in the study will be meaningless. After the reporting of final sample size, authors can describe power analyses, sample size estimations, and confidence level estimations that were calculated to ensure that the study sample size was adequate to yield reliable statistical results. It is important to acknowledge the number of missing items and describe the protocol for handling missing items (*missing items* refers to either the average number of missing items per instrument or the percentage of missing responses per item).

The remainder of the Results section consists of a reporting of your findings and should be organized in accordance with the order of research questions or hypotheses outlined in the purpose section of the Introduction. Findings should be reported for each research question without interpretation. Results should be reported using statistical test and *p* values.

See Chapter 7, Reporting Statistical Data in Text and Tables, to understand how to correctly report statistical tests and symbols in the Results section.

A concisely and well-written Results section should be approximately one to three double-spaced, typed pages in length, depending on the number of psychometric properties addressed in the study.

Discussion

The Discussion section provides the opportunity for authors to interpret findings about the instrument's psychometric properties. It is important that authors not overstate their findings but rather report results with caution and acknowledge study limitations such as sample size insufficiency. Authors should refrain from using exemplars or qualifiers (such as *excellent*) when interpreting the psychometric properties of the assessed instrument. It is more appropriate to use the terms *low*, *moderate*, and *high* and allow readers to independently interpret the numeric values of statistical tests. The Discussion section should be organized in accordance with the research questions or hypotheses stated in the Introduction and Results sections. Authors should answer each research question or hypothesis based on study findings and report whether findings are novel, support previous studies, or challenge previously established information about an instrument's properties and use.

Limitations

In the Limitations subsection, authors should acknowledge the weaknesses of the study that may have biased results. Common limitations in an intervention study include small sample size (that was insufficient for statistical power), use of convenience samples, missing data, compromised blinding procedures, failure to use a panel of experts in content validity studies, and failure to determine that patients remained stable on the construct being measured in the interval between measurements (in reliability studies). Authors should discuss the generalizability of the sample to the larger population and address differences between the target population and the study sample.

Future Research

In the Future Research subsection, authors should suggest ways in which the above limitations can be addressed in more rigorous studies and identify research questions that remain unanswered concerning the instrument's development, refinement, and use with the intended population.

When the Limitations and Future Research subsections are brief, they can be combined into one subheading, *Limitations and Future Research*.

A concisely and well-written Discussion section should be approximately four to five double-spaced, typed pages in length.

Conclusion or Implications for Practice

In this final manuscript section, authors should summarize findings about the instrument's properties and, based on the findings, recommend how the instrument should be used in practice in its present developmental stage. Practitioners and researchers will best benefit from a brief discussion about the instrument's reliable and valid use with specific populations and settings. A concisely, well-written Implications for Practice section should be approximately 250 to 300 words.

After the end of the Implications for Practice section, the following are the remaining manuscript sections in the order in which they should be presented in the paper:

- References
- Tables
- Figures

CHECKLIST FOR MANUSCRIPT STRUCTURE AND CONTENT OF INSTRUMENT DEVELOPMENT AND TESTING STUDIES

Title

☐ Include the following: population, instrument name or construct measured, psychometric properties assessed.

Abstract

☐ Objectives: In one to two sentences, describe the purpose of the study, which will address the development or further refinement of an instrument and/or the assessment of its psychometric properties.

☐ Method: In one to two sentences, provide information about the research design, study time line, participants (population, sample size), and data collection procedures.

☐ Results: In one to two sentences, report the primary findings along with statistical test results as calculated using either CTT or IRT.

☐ Conclusions: In one to two sentences, describe the implications of findings for the instrument's use with the targeted population.

Introduction

☐ Describe the background of the problem as it relates to the population, profession, and society.

☐ Report the incidence of the targeted population.

☐ Describe the impact of the diagnosis or clinical problem on functional community participation.

☐ Define the construct measured by the instrument.

☐ Define all novel or unfamiliar terms directly when first mentioned.

☐ Discuss the literature examining how the construct has been measured in the targeted population using other instruments.

☐ Describe the need for the instrument.

☐ Provide a brief description of the instrument (a detailed description will be made in the Method section).

☐ Describe the theoretical base for an instrument that is newly developed.

☐ Purpose statement: detail the need to establish specific psychometric properties for the instrument.

☐ Provide precise research questions or a priori hypotheses (include the direction and magnitude of expectations for all hypotheses).

Method

Research Design

☐ Indicate the specific type of research design used (beyond stating that the study is a psychometric study).

- State and define the specific types of reliability and/or validity that were assessed.
- Indicate whether the design is based on CTT or IRT.
- Indicate whether retrospective or prospective data have been collected.
- Indicate whether institutional review board or ethics committee approval was obtained or exempted.
- Indicate whether participants provided consent.

Participants

- Describe the sampling method and setting(s) from which participants were selected.
- Describe the inclusion and exclusion criteria so that readers can understand the characteristics of the target population.

Instruments

- Describe the instrument with regard to purpose, intended population, type of data collected (e.g., self-report, performance based observer rating, Likert scale, open-ended questions, or total score yielding ratio data), and administration length and setting.
- Provide information about previously established psychometric properties regarding reliability, validity, and responsiveness (provide citations for all psychometric studies).
- When convergent and criterion validity are assessed, the comparison instrument should be described in detail with regard to the above information.

Procedures

- Document the process of instrument development, revision, or translation.
- Document the procedures through which reliability, validity, and/or responsiveness were assessed.
- Detail the study timeline and sequence of events.
- Describe the setting in which instrument administration occurred.

Content Validity

- Indicate whether an assessment was performed to determine the following:
  - Whether all test items refer to relevant aspects of the construct and collectively reflect the construct
  - Whether all items are relevant for the study population with regard to age, gender, disease characteristics, geographical region or country, setting
  - Whether a table of specifications was used to determine the number, range, and content of instrument items
  - Whether a panel of content experts was used to assess content validity

Convergent and Criterion Validity

- Document the steps used to ensure that the comparison instrument was a reasonable gold standard or best available instrument for comparison.
- Indicate whether evaluators were blinded to the other measures to minimize the risk of expectation and limit biased ratings.

Reliability

☐ For assessment of reliability including interrater, intrarater, and test-retest, report the following:

  ○ Whether at least two measurements were available for comparison

  ○ Whether the instrument administrations were independent of each other—the first administration did not influence the second

  ○ The time interval between instrument administrations (2 weeks is customary for most reliability studies and is considered long enough to reduce the risk of item recall but short enough to limit the possibility that the patient did not maintain stability on the construct being measured)

  ○ Whether patients were stable on the construct measured over the 2-week period of instrument administration

  ○ Whether conditions were the same for both instrument administrations (i.e., setting, type of instructions provided)

  ○ For interrater reliability, whether raters were blinded to each other's scores to reduce bias

☐ For internal consistency, report whether scale unidimensionality was checked.

Translation Studies

☐ When an instrument has been translated into another language, indicate the following:

  ○ The expertise level of the translators with regard to language translation, knowledge of the diagnosis, and knowledge of the construct measured by the instrument

  ○ Whether the translators worked independently of each other

  ○ Whether back and forward translation were performed

  ○ How differences between the original and translated instrument versions were resolved

  ○ Whether the translation was reviewed by a panel of experts

  ○ Whether the translated instrument was pretested to check for possible problems in interpretation, cultural relevance, and understandability

Data Collection

☐ Report the data collection schedule with regard to the sequence of data collection and how and by whom data were collected.

☐ Describe data collectors with regard to type of professional, expertise level, and training in data collection procedures.

☐ In convergent and criterion validity studies, indicate whether data collectors were blinded to the other instrument and participant scores to reduce expectation bias.

☐ In interrater reliability studies, indicate whether data collectors were blinded to each other's scores.

Data Analysis

☐ Report whether data analysis was based on CTT or IRT.

☐ For CTT:

  ○ Describe and cite all statistical test methods.

  ○ Justify and cite the use of nontraditional statistical procedures that are incongruent with traditional parametric and nonparametric data analysis.

- Justify and cite the use of statistical tests that may be congruent with traditional parametric and nonparametric data analysis but are likely unfamiliar to readers.
- Identify and cite the software program used to generate statistical analysis.
- Indicate at what significance level probability was set.

- For IRT:
  - Describe the IRT model used (e.g., one-parameter logistic model, OPLM; partial credit model, PCM; graded response model, GRM).
  - Name and cite the software program used (e.g., RUMM2020, WINSTEPS, OPLM, MULTILOG, PARSCALE, BILOG, NLMIXED).
  - Report the method of estimation used (e.g., conditional maximum likelihood, CML; marginal maximum likelihood, MML).
  - Identify the assumptions for estimating parameters of the IRT model (unidimensionality; local independence; and item fit, differential item functioning or DIF).

Results

- Provide the final sample size.
- Report information about the number of participants who withdrew because they could not tolerate test conditions (and why).
- Report participant demographics with regard to age, gender, race, ethnicity, education level, socioeconomic level, and topic-specific characteristics such as functional status.
- Describe power analyses, sample size estimations, and confidence level estimations that were calculated to ensure that the study sample size was adequate to yield reliable statistical results.
- Acknowledge the number of missing items and describe the protocol for handling missing items.
- Organize and report findings in accordance with the order of research questions or hypotheses outlined in the Introduction section.
- Report results using statistical test and p values.

Discussion

- Organize and provide interpretations of findings in accordance with the order of research questions or hypotheses outlined in the Results section.
- Be cautious not to overstate findings.
- Indicate whether findings are novel, support previous studies, or challenge previously established information about an instrument's properties and use.

Limitations

- Acknowledge limitations such as small sample size, use of convenience samples, missing data, compromised blinding procedures, failure to use a panel of experts in content validity studies, and failure to determine that patients remained stable on the construct being measured in the interval between measurements (in reliability studies).
- Discuss the generalizability of the sample to the larger population and address differences between the target population and the study sample.

Future Research

- ☐ Suggest ways in which limitations can be addressed in more rigorous studies.
- ☐ Identify research questions that remain unanswered concerning the instrument's development, refinement, and use with the intended population.

Conclusion or Implications for Practice

- ☐ Summarize findings about the instrument's properties.
- ☐ Suggest how the instrument should be used in practice in its present developmental stage.

EXAMPLES OF WELL-WRITTEN INSTRUMENT DEVELOPMENT AND TESTING ARTICLES

Classen, S., Wang, Y., Winter, S. M., Velozo, C. A., Lanford, D. N., & Bédard, M. (2013). Concurrent criterion validity of the Safe Driving Behavior Measure: A predictor of on-road driving outcomes. *American Journal of Occupational Therapy, 67*(1), 108–116. doi:10.5014/ajot.2013.005116

Hwang, J. E. (2012). Development and validation of a 15-item Lifestyle Screening for Community Dwelling Older Adults. *American Journal of Occupational Therapy, 66*, e98–e106. doi:10.5014/ajot.2012.005181

Ohl, A., Butler, C., Carney, C., Jarmel, E., Palmierie, M., Pottheiser, D., & Smith, T. (2012). Test-retest reliability of the Sensory Profile Caregiver Questionnaire. *American Journal of Occupational Therapy, 66*(4), 483–487. doi:10.5014/ajot.2012.003517

REFERENCES

American Psychological Association. (2010). *Publication manual of the American Psychological Association* (6th ed.). Washington, DC: Author.

Mokkink, L. B., Terwee, C. B., Patrick, D. L., Alonso, J., Stratford, P. W., Knol, D. L., . . . de Vet, H. C. (2010). The COSMIN study reached international consensus on taxonomy, terminology, and definitions of measurement properties for health-related patient-reported outcomes. *Journal of Clinical Epidemiology, 63*(7), 737–745. doi:10.1016/j.jclinepi.2010.02.006

6

Manuscript Structure and Content for Case Reports

A case report is a type of manuscript design in which the results of one patient's response to a novel intervention is reported, usually by the treating health care professional. Case reports were originally designed for physicians to describe treatment and outcomes of one patient in response to a novel treatment method but have been adopted by other health professionals. Traditional case reports do not require the rigor of manualized intervention or written treatment guidelines (because treatment protocols are in the early stages of development), the use of instruments with established psychometric properties, baseline and postintervention measures, and statistical analysis of data. The CARE Statement (Gagnier et al., 2013) provides a template and checklist for traditional case report writing.

In the effort to build evidence supporting health care intervention methods, I recommend that case reports be made more rigorous by the addition of preliminary written protocols, the use of instruments with strong psychometric properties, baseline and postintervention measures, basic statistical analysis of data when possible, and qualitative data describing the patient or client's perception of intervention. I additionally recommend that authors use the following structure and content for case report writing.

MANUSCRIPT HEADINGS FOR CASE REPORTS

The following heading levels are based on American Psychological Association (2010) formatting.

Title

(Begin the manuscript with a title on a separate title page. The title should be centered and typed in uppercase and lowercase letters.)

Gutman, S. A. *Journal Article Writing and Publication: Your Guide to Mastering Clinical Health Care Reporting Standards* (pp. 51-62).© 2017 Taylor & Francis Group.

Abstract

(The Abstract should be placed on the page directly following the title page. The word *Abstract* should be capitalized and centered.)

Introduction

(The Introduction begins on the page directly following the abstract. The heading *Introduction* is not typed in the manuscript because the beginning of the manuscript text alerts the reader that the Introduction has begun.)

Method

(The Method section is positioned directly after the Introduction. The heading *Method* is centered and bolded.)

Case Report Design

(*Case Report Design* is the first subheading in the Method section. It is bolded and flush left).

Participant Selection and History

(*Participant Selection and History* is the second subheading in the Method section. It is bolded and flush left.)

Instruments (or Outcome Measures)

(*Instruments,* or *Outcome Measures,* is the third subheading in the Method section. It is bolded and flush left.)

Intervention

(*Intervention* is the fourth subheading in the Method sections. It is bolded and flush left.)

Intervention description.
(*Intervention description* is the first subheading of the Intervention subsection. It is indented, bolded, and ends with a period. Only the first letter of the first word is capitalized. The manuscript text begins directly after the period.)

Interveners.
(*Interveners,* or *Interventionists,* is the second subheading of the Intervention subsection. It is indented, bolded, and ends with a period. The *I* in Interveners is capitalized. The manuscript text begins directly after the period.)

Intervention fidelity.
(*Intervention fidelity* is the third subheading of the Intervention subsection. It is indented, bolded, and ends with a period. Only the first letter of the first word is capitalized. The manuscript text begins directly after the period.)

Data Collection

(*Data Collection* is the subheading that directly follows Intervention fidelity. It is bolded and flush left.)

Data Analysis

(*Data Analysis* is the subheading that directly follows Data Collection. It is bolded and flush left.)

Results

(The Results section directly follows Data Analysis and begins a new section of the paper. The heading *Results* is bolded and centered.)

Discussion

(The Discussion section directly follows the Results section and begins a new section of the paper. The heading *Discussion* is bolded and centered.)

Limitations

(The Limitations subsection is part of the Discussion section but should be highlighted for the reader by a separate subheading within the Discussion section. The subheading *Limitations* is bolded and flush left.)

Future Research

(The Future Research section directly follows the Limitations subsection. This section is also part of the Discussion section and should be highlighted for the reader by a separate subheading label. The subheading *Future Research* is bolded and flush left.)

Conclusion or Implications for Practice

(The Conclusion section, also labeled Implications for Practice, is often the final section of a manuscript. It is a new manuscript section directly following the Discussion section. The heading is bolded and centered.)

References

(References begin on a separate page following the Conclusion. The heading is centered and not bolded.)

Tables

(Tables should be provided after the end of the references and begin on a separate page. Each table should be presented on its own page. Tables are named and presented in accordance with the order in which they are mentioned in the text.)

Figures

(Figures should be provided after the end of the tables and begin on a separate page. Each figure should be presented on its own page. Figures are named and presented in accordance with the order in which they are mentioned in the text.)

MANUSCRIPT LENGTH

A case report should be approximately 4,000 to 5,000 words in length (including references). The length of a case report should be shorter than a feature-length manuscript reporting an intervention effectiveness study. Authors should refer to a specific journal's author guidelines to determine page length and word count for case reports.

MANUSCRIPT HEADING CONTENT FOR CASE REPORTS

There should be no repetition of content in the manuscript. The sections and subsections mentioned next should not contain overlap and will not if written as suggested.

Title

Case report titles should contain four essential elements to help indexers categorize the article so that it can be easily accessed by the intended audience.

1. The patient's diagnosis and age group

2. The intervention (the independent variable)

3. The outcome measures (the dependent variable)

4. The words *case report* (the research design)

Examples of good case report titles include the following:

- Effect of a Social Skills Program on the Communication of a Nonverbal Adolescent With Autism: A Case Report

- Effect of Occupational Therapy Services on the Housing Transition of a Homeless Man With Psychiatric Disability and Substance Abuse: A Case Report

- A Case Report of Sensory Integration Therapy for a Child With Obsessive Compulsive Disorder

Abbreviations in the title should be avoided unless commonly used and understood in the health care community.

Abstract

Abstracts for case reports are written similarly to those for intervention effectiveness studies and are best organized by use of the following headings, unless indicated otherwise by a specific journal's author guidelines: (a) objectives, (b) method, (c) results, and (d) conclusions. Addressing each subheading above—and the specific content that belongs in each subheading—will ensure that you provide editors, reviewers, and readers with essential information about the intervention, patient or client, method, and findings. Because readers select papers primarily based on abstracts, the provision of this essential information is critical for the transparent reporting of case reports. Although most case report abstracts are between 150 and 200 words in length, authors are advised to check a specific journal's author guidelines and adhere to the stated word count.

- Objectives: In one to two sentences, authors should describe the purpose of the study. In a case report, the study purpose will address the initial assessment of a novel intervention for a specific patient or client.

- Method: In one to two sentences, authors should provide information about the patient or client (diagnosis, age group, functional status, etc.), setting, research design (e.g., case report with pre- and posttest measures), intervention length and description, follow-up points if any, and outcome measures.

- Results: In one to two sentences, authors should report findings about the intervention's effect (if used, statistical test results and *p* values should be reported) and the patient's perceptions of intervention.

- Conclusions: In one to two sentences, authors should (a) describe the implications of the intervention for the patient's functional status and independence and (b) address how these preliminary findings can be used to inform future research and practice.

Introduction

The Introduction of a case report should be no longer than four double-spaced, typed pages. Similar to intervention effectiveness studies, the Introduction of case reports should provide background information about the problem as it relates to the patient, profession, and society.

Information about the patient diagnosis (relating to incidence and functional independence in the community) should be provided along with a discussion of traditional interventions (and their effectiveness) used to address the problems associated with the diagnosis. The need for the novel intervention examined in the present study should be justified for the reader and the intervention should be briefly described; a detailed description of the intervention will be provided in the Method section. Authors should discuss the theoretical basis for the novel intervention and describe any previous intervention studies that report similar treatment approaches. If no intervention studies reporting similar approaches exist, authors must clearly state this. The 5-year rule for citation use should be applied; however, when more recent literature does not exist, articles with publication dates of more than 5 years can be used to discuss the theoretical base, traditionally used interventions for this diagnosis, and studies of similar treatment approaches. Articles about incidence should not be older than 2 to 3 years.

The purpose statement is the final paragraph of the Introduction. Here, authors should state the purpose of the present case report and provide clear and precise research questions. Research questions for a case report should contain the patient diagnosis and age group, intervention, and outcome measures. The research questions should clearly indicate that the research design involves one patient or client. If research questions were not formally developed at the outset of treatment, authors can discuss the clinical hypotheses that supported their decision to administer intervention.

Examples of good case report research questions include the following:

- Can a client-centered, sensory-based, nutritional diet decrease food refusal in a child with autism spectrum disorder?

- Can a robotic device increase upper extremity use of an adult with hemiplegia 1 month after stroke?

- Can a housing and life skills program help a homeless man to transition from a shelter to supportive housing and maintain housing at 6-month follow-up?

Definitions

All new and unfamiliar terms that are presented in the Introduction (and throughout the text) should be defined when the term first appears in the manuscript. Common mistakes include failing to define terms, unclearly defining terms, presenting terms in one section and defining them in another, and changing the definition of a term within a paper. To understand how to write a good definition, authors should see Chapter 3, p. 13.

Quotations

As stated in Chapters 3, 4, and 5, quotations should only be used in scholarly writing when quoting a historical source or legal document; presenting a specific definition accepted by the scientific community, whose meaning would change if the exact wording were altered; and verbatim responses from patients or clients. With the exception of these instances, quotations should be avoided in health care writing. Instead, paraphrase and cite the original source.

A concisely and well-written Introduction should be approximately three to four double-spaced, typed pages in length.

Method

The Method section of a case report details your selection of a patient or client for the novel intervention, collection of baseline measures, intervention administration, collection of posttest measures, and analysis of findings. The Method section must provide specific details about the above so that (a) researchers can replicate findings and design larger studies; (b) practitioners can determine if the intervention may have potential benefit for their own patients; and (c) editors, reviewers, and readers can evaluate the rigor of the case report. The use of the following subheadings in the Method section, and the content belonging in each subheading, will help you provide transparent and essential information.

Case Report Design

The case report design, or the sequence of treatment and data collection, should be explained in this section. For example:

- Pretest/posttest design with 3-month follow-up
- Baseline data collection, first intervention period, first postintervention data collection, second intervention period, second postintervention data collection

In addition to the sequence of treatment and data collection, authors should indicate whether the patient provided consent for his or her data to be used in future publication (authors should ethically attempt to obtain patient consent either during treatment or after discharge once the decision has been made to use patient data for a case report). Authors should also state whether their use of patient data in the case report was exempted or approved by an institutional review board or ethics committee. Many institutional review boards will exempt data collected during health care practice; however, such exemption must be sought and then declared in the case report.

Participant Selection and History

Authors must describe the setting from which the patient was selected to receive the novel treatment, the patient characteristics that designated him or her as a good candidate for the novel intervention, and the patient's health history. Minimal reporting standards require that patient demographics include age, gender, race, ethnicity, and socioeconomic status. Functional status and level of independence in community participation should also be addressed. Transparent reporting standards require that the health professional who selected the patient for intervention, and the relationship of that person to the patient, be disclosed in this section.

Instruments (or Outcome Measures)

All instruments and outcome measures (such as frequency counts of specific behaviors) used to gather baseline and postintervention data should be described and cited in this section. Detailed descriptions of all instruments will allow readers to evaluate whether the selected instruments were appropriate to measure the targeted outcomes. Instruments (including clinical assessment tools such as goniometers, edema volumeters, and dynamometers) should be described with regard to purpose, intended population, type of data collected (e.g., self-report, performance based observer rating, Likert scale, open-ended questions, or total score yielding ratio data), and administration length. Psychometric properties of each instrument should be provided in numeric value, with statistical test and p values indicated (all psychometric properties should be cited). If authors have used an instrument without established psychometric properties or if an instrument has been newly developed for this case report, this information must be clearly stated in this section. Using instruments without established reliability and validity may yield questionable findings, and authors should justify their decision to use such an instrument. Frequency counts of desired behaviors (or other clinically targeted outcomes), however, do not require reliability and validity data and are appropriate for case reports. If authors have developed an assessment for this case report to measure a specific outcome, they should describe the development process and disclose if procedures included the evaluation of face or content validity through an expert panel. The provision of sample items in a table or figure will help readers understand whether the newly developed instrument targets the examined outcome measure for which it was designed.

Intervention

The Intervention section is unique to intervention effectiveness studies and case reports and is divided into the following three subsections:

1. *Intervention description.* The intervention should be described with regard to the following:
   - The number and length of sessions (dosage) and the length of the intervention over time (duration)
   - The content of each session
   - Whether intervention was delivered individually or in a group

   The clinical course should be described including any interruption in or discontinuation of treatment. Authors should disclose whether the patient received any type of simultaneous clinical service that could not be controlled and whose influence may have affected results.

2. *Interveners.* Information about those providing intervention should detail the following:
   - The type of professional(s) who provided treatment
   - The number of therapists involved in care
   - The type and length of training that the therapist(s) received to administer intervention

3. *Intervention fidelity.* Intervention fidelity refers to the procedures used to ensure that the intervention was both administered in accordance with a written manual and uniformly if multiple interveners delivered intervention. In case report designs, it is common that written manuals have not as yet been developed. If multiple interveners were involved in care delivery, however, there should be some method to ensure that all therapists provided intervention uniformly. When multiple interveners are involved, authors should describe the procedures used to assess intervention fidelity or conversely, state clearly that intervention fidelity was not evaluated.

Data Collection

In a case report, it is common for the treating therapist to collect data; however, such overlap of roles should be clearly stated because this condition may introduce bias and influence results. Authors should describe how, when, and by whom each set of data was collected. If multiple data collectors were used, authors should detail how data collectors were trained to collect data uniformly and whether interrater reliability was established.

Data Analysis

All descriptive, statistical, and qualitative data analysis methods used to compare baseline and postintervention measures, and analyze the patient's perceptions of treatment, should be described and cited. Statistical analysis that will likely be unfamiliar to readers or is incongruent with traditional parametric and nonparametric data analysis rules should be justified and cited. Similarly, descriptive and qualitative methods used to understand the patient's response to treatment should be described and cited. The names and citations of all analytic software programs should also be provided, and the level at which statistical significance was set for quantitative tests should be reported.

A concisely and well-written Method section should be approximately three to four double-spaced, typed pages in length.

Results

The Results section in a case report (a) details the findings on baseline, postintervention, and follow-up measures; and (b) documents the patient's perception of intervention on self-report measures and qualitative interviews. The patient's intervention experience should include information about satisfaction, congruence with cultural values, and ability to help the patient attain personal health goals. Family member and caregiver reports may also be used to provide supplemental information in addition to the patient's responses, particularly when patients may experience cognitive disorders that limit or alter perception or when children are participants. Authors should aim to supplement quantitative and qualitative data with information about gains the patient has made in postintervention functional community participation based on patient, family member, caregiver, and teacher, etc., reports. The Results section should be organized in accordance with the order of research questions outlined in the purpose statement (of the Introduction). Findings should be reported for each research question. While the provision of raw scores is not typical in intervention effectiveness studies with multiple participants, raw score reporting in tables and figures is customary in a case report. When statistical analysis has been performed to compare baseline and postintervention measures, the statistical test and p values should be reported. Qualitative data may be supported by quotations from the patient, family member, or caregiver. Authors should also document the occurrence of any adverse effects or unexpected findings.

See Chapter 7, Reporting Statistical Data in Text and Tables, to clarify how to correctly report statistical tests and symbols in the Results section.

A concisely and well-written Results section should be approximately three double-spaced, typed pages in length.

Discussion

The Discussion section in a case report allows authors to interpret the findings reported in the Results section as they relate to the patient. It is important that authors do not overstate their findings about the intervention's effectiveness because case reports lack the rigor of control, randomization, larger sample sizes, and blinding procedures. In a case report, authors can only state that the intervention appeared to be effective with the participating patient. While generalization of findings cannot be made, authors can suggest that the intervention shows promise and warrants future study with larger sample sizes and more rigorous study methods. The Discussion section should be organized according to the order of research questions (or hypotheses) provided in the purpose statement and addressed in the Results section. Authors should attempt to answer each research question based on findings presented in the Results section. Unanticipated findings should be explained, and the occurrence of adverse events should be examined with regard to intervention risk and safety. Authors should discuss how the case report findings can contribute to the body of research needed to build consensus regarding best practice.

Limitations

A case report has inherent weaknesses in internal and external validity that should be documented in the Limitations section.

Weaknesses in internal validity (i.e., the degree to which researchers can be confident that the changes in outcome measures were a result of the intervention) include the following:

- Possible lack of intervention fidelity if multiple interveners were used or failure to assess intervention fidelity
- Compromised blinding of the intervener(s) and data collector(s)
- Insufficient sample size power
- Lack of control and randomization
- Possible use of instruments with little or no established psychometric properties

Weaknesses in external validity (i.e., the degree to which researchers can be confident that the participants represent the larger population) include the following:

- Possible influence of participant incentives
- One patient's findings cannot be generalized to the larger population

If follow-up points were not incorporated into the case report design, a further weakness would involve the inability to understand whether gains made as a possible result of intervention lasted over time.

Future Research

In the Future Research section, authors can recommend future study designs that address the previously-noted limitations.

Because the separate subsections Limitations and Future Research are often brief, authors may combine them into one subheading, *Limitations and Future Research.*

A concisely and well-written Discussion section should be approximately four double-spaced, typed pages in length.

Conclusion or Implications for Practice

In this final section of a case report, authors should summarize the major study findings and describe how these findings have potential to contribute to future research and practice.

After the end of the Implications for Practice, the following are the remaining manuscript sections in the order in which they should be presented in the paper:

- References
- Tables
- Figures

CHECKLIST FOR MANUSCRIPT CONTENT AND STRUCTURE OF CASE REPORTS

Title

☐ Include the following elements: patient diagnosis and age group, intervention, outcome measures, case report.

Abstract

☐ Objectives: In one to two sentences, describe the purpose of the study. In a case report, the study purpose will address the initial assessment of a novel intervention for a specific patient or client.

☐ Method: In one to two sentences, provide information about the patient or client (diagnosis, age group, functional status, etc.), setting, research design (e.g., case report with pre- and posttest measures), intervention length and description, follow-up points if any, and outcome measures.

☐ Results: In one to two sentences, authors should report findings about the intervention's effect (if used, statistical test results and *p* values should be reported) and the patient's perceptions of intervention.

☐ Conclusions: In one to two sentences, authors should (a) describe the implications of the intervention for the patient's functional status and independence and (b) address how these preliminary findings can be used to inform future research and practice.

Introduction

☐ Provide background information about the problem as it relates to the patient, profession, and society.

□ Provide information about the patient diagnosis relating to incidence and functional independence in the community.

□ Discuss traditional interventions (and their effectiveness) used to address the problems associated with the diagnosis.

□ Justify the need for the novel intervention.

□ Briefly describe the intervention.

□ Discuss the intervention's theoretical base.

□ Purpose statement: state the purpose of the present case report.

□ Research questions: provide clear and precise research questions that contain patient diagnosis and age group, intervention, and outcome measures. Indicate that only one patient is involved.

□ If research questions were not formally developed at the outset of treatment, discuss clinical hypotheses.

□ Make sure that all terms are well defined as soon as they are presented in the manuscript.

Method

Case Report Design

□ Describe the case report design or sequence of treatment and data collection.

□ Indicate whether patient consent was obtained.

□ Indicate whether institutional review board or ethics committee approval or exemption was obtained.

Participant Selection and History

□ Describe the setting from which the patient was selected, patient characteristics, and patient health history.

□ Describe patient demographics including age, gender, race, ethnicity, and socioeconomic status.

□ Describe functional status and level of independence in community participation.

□ Identify the person who selected the patient for intervention and that person's relationship to the patient.

Instruments (or Outcome Measures)

□ Describe, and cite, all instruments and outcome measures used to gather baseline and postintervention data with regard to purpose, intended population, type of data collected, and administration length.

□ Provide the psychometric properties for each instrument in numeric value, with statistical test and p values indicated; provide citations for all established psychometric properties. Disclose if no established psychometric properties exist.

□ If an assessment has been newly developed for this case report, describe the development process. Provide sample items in tables or figures.

Intervention

Intervention Description

□ Describe the number and length of sessions (dosage) and the length of the intervention over time (duration), the content of each session, and whether intervention was delivered individually or in a group.

- ▫ Describe the clinical course including any interruption in or discontinuation of treatment.
- ▫ Disclose if the patient received any type of simultaneous clinical service that could not be controlled and whose influence may have affected results.

Interveners

- ▫ Describe the type of professional(s) who provided treatment, the number of therapists involved in care, and the type and length of training that the therapist(s) received to administer intervention.

Intervention Fidelity

- ▫ When multiple interveners are involved, authors should describe the procedures used to assess intervention fidelity or conversely, state clearly that intervention fidelity was not evaluated.

Data Collection

- ▫ Describe how, when, and by whom each set of data was collected.
- ▫ Disclose if the intervener also collected data.
- ▫ If multiple data collectors were used, detail how data collectors were trained to collect data uniformly and whether interrater reliability was established.

Data Analysis

- ▫ Describe and cite all descriptive, statistical, and qualitative data analysis methods used to compare baseline and postintervention measures and analyze the patient's perceptions of treatment.
- ▫ Justify and cite statistical analysis that will likely be unfamiliar to readers or is incongruent with traditional parametric and nonparametric data analysis rules.
- ▫ Describe and cite qualitative methods used to understand the patient's response to treatment.
- ▫ Identify and cite all analytic software programs used and the level at which statistical significance was set for quantitative tests.

Results

- ▫ Detail the findings on baseline, postintervention, and follow-up measures.
- ▫ Document the patient's perception of intervention on self-report measures and qualitative interviews.
- ▫ Supplement quantitative and qualitative data with information about gains the patient made in postintervention functional community participation.
- ▫ Organize the Results section in accordance with the order of research questions outlined in the purpose statement (of the Introduction). Findings should be reported for each research question.
- ▫ When statistical analysis has been performed to compare baseline and postintervention measures, the statistical test and *p* values should be reported.
- ▫ Support qualitative findings with quotations from the patient or family member or caregiver.
- ▫ Report any adverse effects or unexpected findings.

Discussion

- ▫ Be careful not to overstate findings or generalize results beyond the patient.

- Organize the Discussion section according to the order of research questions (or hypotheses) provided in the purpose statement and addressed in the Results section.
- Explain unanticipated findings.
- Discuss adverse events as they relate to intervention safety and risk.
- Discuss how the case report findings can contribute to the body of research needed to build consensus regarding best practice.

Limitations

- Discuss weaknesses in internal validity with regard to the following:
  - Possible lack of intervention fidelity if multiple interveners were used or failure to assess intervention fidelity
  - Compromised blinding of the intervener(s) and data collector(s)
  - Insufficient sample size power
  - Lack of control and randomization
  - Possible use of instruments with little or no established psychometric properties
- Discuss weaknesses in external validity with regard to the use of one participant and the possible influence of participant incentives.

Future Research

- Recommend future study designs that address the above-noted limitations.

Conclusion or Implications for Practice

- Summarize the major study findings and describe how these findings have potential to contribute to future research and practice.

EXAMPLES OF WELL-WRITTEN CASE REPORTS

Gutman, S. A., Raphael-Greenfield, E. I., Kerr, L., Siedlitz, E., & Wang, C. (2014). Using motor-based role-play to enhance social skills in a nonverbal adolescent with high functioning autism: A case report. *Occupational Therapy in Mental Health, 30,* 12–25. doi:10.1080/0164212X.2014.878235

Nilsen, D. M., & DiRusso, T. (2014). Using mirror therapy in the home environment: A case report. *American Journal of Occupational Therapy, 68,* e84–e89. doi:10.5014/ajot.2014.010389

REFERENCES

American Psychological Association. (2010). *Publication manual of the American Psychological Association* (6th ed.). Washington, DC: Author.

Gagnier, J. J., Kienle, G., Altman, D. G., Moher, D., Sox, H., & Riley, D., for the CARE Group. (2013). The CARE Guidelines: Consensus-based clinical case reporting guideline development. *Global Advances in Health and Medicine, 2*(5), 38–43. doi:10.7453/gahmj.2013.008

7

Reporting Statistical Data in Text and Tables

Correctly preparing a research manuscript involves the appropriate reporting of numbers, statistics, symbols, and mathematical copy in text and tables. Inappropriate reporting of these items can adversely influence an editor's, reviewer's, and reader's perception of a manuscript's quality. There are numerous rules guiding the reporting of numbers and statistical data detailed in the *Publication Manual of the American Psychological Association,* 6th ed. (American Psychological Association, 2010). Rather than duplicate this information, this section aims to review the most commonly used rules and help authors avoid frequently made mistakes.

NUMBERS

The general rule for the reporting of numbers in the manuscript text is to use numerals for numbers 10 and above; numbers below 10 should be spelled out. There are the following exceptions to this rule, however:

- Numbers that immediately precede a unit of measurement should be written in numeric form.
  - 5 mm, 1 in, 6 lbs
- Numbers that represent statistical or mathematical functions, percentages, ratios, decimals, and fractions should be written in numeric form.
  - 7% of the population
  - More males than females have a diagnosis of ASD at a ratio of 4:1
  - The 3rd percentile
  - 4 times as many adults

Gutman, S. A. *Journal Article Writing and Publication: Your Guide to Mastering Clinical Health Care Reporting Standards* (pp. 63-67). © 2017 Taylor & Francis Group.

- Numbers that represent time, dates, age, and exact monetary sums should be written in numeric form.
  - The test takes 1 hour to administer.
  - The second phase began at 3:00 pm.
  - The patient was 8 years old.
  - Participants were given $5 as an incentive.
  Exception: When approximating the number of days, months, and years, spell out numbers.
  - The participant had a biopsy approximately two months ago.
- Numbers that represent scores or points on an instrument scale should be written in numeric form.
  - Participant B scored 5 on a 20-point scale.
- Numbers that indicate a place in a series should be written in numeric form.
  - The students were in grade 5.
  - The instruments were set out on table 3.
  - The participants were at reading level 6.
- Numbers that begin a sentence, title, or heading should always be spelled out.
  - Thirty-three percent of the population experiences anxiety.
  - Fifteen students were selected to participate.
- Common fractions in a sentence should be spelled out.
  - One third of the class scored at the highest percentile.
  - Two-thirds of our participants had concomitant disorders.

NUMBERS EXPRESSED AS PLURALS

Numbers in plural form are indicated by adding *s* or *es* to the numeral or word without an apostrophe.
- 1960s
- 50s and 100s
- Sixes, sevens, and eights

DECIMALS

When writing decimals in the text and in tables use the following rules:
- When the statistic can exceed 1, use a zero before the decimal point.
  - $t = 0.24$
  - $d = 0.14$
- When the statistic cannot exceed 1, do not use a zero before the decimal point.
  - $p = .05$
  - $r = .68$

- For probability levels, report decimals to two or three places.
  - $p = .027$
  - $p < .001$
  - $p < .05$
- Round all other decimals reported in the text and tables to two decimal places.
  - $t = 0.58$
  - $r = .74$

STATISTICAL SYMBOLS

When writing statistical letters expressed as symbols in text and tables, use the following rules:
- Letters used to indicate the names of statistical tests should be italicized.
  - $F(1, 33) = 4.43, p = .04$
  - $t = 2.28, p = .032$, 95% CI [.75, .95]
- Use the word, instead of the symbol, when reporting a statistical term in a narrative sentence, but not within parentheses.
  - The mean age was 55 (not the M age was 55).
  - Participants ranged in age from 45-65 ($M = 55$, $SD = 10$).

SYMBOLS FOR NUMBER OF PARTICIPANTS

- An upper case, italicized N should be used to indicate the total number of participants for a sample.
  - $N = 50$
- A lowercase, italicized n is used to indicate the number of participants in a sample subgroup.
  - $n = 15$

PERCENT SYMBOL

- Use the percent symbol when it is preceded by a numeral.
  - 18%
- When a percentage is not preceded by a numeral, spell the word.
  - The percentage of adults with ADHD is anticipated to be higher than thought.
- Use the percent symbol, %, in table headings and figure legends to conserve space.
  - Correlation Between School Drop-Out and % of Students Using Alcohol

SPACING OF STATISTICAL AND NUMERICAL SYMBOLS

Space statistical and numerical symbols as words with typed intervals between symbols and numerals.

- $t = 2.28$, $p = .032$, 95% CI [.75, .95]
- $F(1, 99) = 6.83$, $p = .006$, 95% CI [.14, .59]

REPORTING STATISTICAL TEST FINDINGS IN THE RESULTS SECTION

The Results section should contain a reporting of findings in both narrative and statistical symbols and numerals.

- An independent t test found a statistically significant difference between intervention and control groups at 1 month after intervention with a moderate effect size ($t = 3.25$, $p = .023$, $d = 0.54$, 95% CI [.12, 73]). The difference between intervention and control group scores at 6 months after intervention was also statistically significant with a larger effect size ($t = 4.88$, $p = .003$, $d = .89$).

REPORTING STATISTICAL TEST FINDINGS IN TABLES

Statistical data reported in the Results narrative should not be duplicated in tables. Tables show numerical values and text in ordered columns and rows and should be used to present a large amount of data that can only be summarized in the Results narrative. Tables should supplement the Results narrative and provide the data necessary for readers to evaluate the researcher's findings using the study's data set. For example, data such as participant mean scores and standard deviations for several instruments could be efficiently displayed in a table without having to use space in the Results narrative.

Authors should refer to all tables in the Results narrative.

- "Table 1 shows participant mean scores and standard deviations for each performance measure."
- "Participant mean scores indicate that as a group, participant performance was highest on the Global Motor Assessment (see Table 1)."

Tables should be numbered according to the order in which they are referred to in the text.

- Tables begin with "1" and are numbered consecutively.
- Suffixes (Table 5a and 5b) are not used.

Tables should be edited with precision, and visual characteristics should be precise, clear, and easy to understand.

- Make sure that table information matches that reported in the manuscript abstract and text— such as final sample size, sample size of subgroups, and reported statistics.
- Make sure that table column numbers and percentages add up correctly.

Inconsistencies between the manuscript text and tables reflect poorly on manuscript quality.

The American Psychological Association (2010) provides extensive information about table formatting, and I encourage authors to review this information when preparing manuscript tables.

Many journals have a limit on the amount of tables that can be submitted in one manuscript, and authors should check a journal's author guidelines to determine table requirements.

REFERENCE

American Psychological Association. (2010). *Publication manual of the American Psychological Association* (6th ed.). Washington, DC: Author.

8

Preparing and Submitting Manuscripts for Publication

All journals have author guidelines that provide instructions for the preparation and submission of manuscripts. Readers are encouraged to obtain and adhere to the guidelines of the specific journal to which they wish to submit at an early stage in the manuscript development process. This section helps readers understand the process of preparing manuscripts for submission and publication.

AUTHORSHIP AND CORRESPONDING AUTHOR RESPONSIBILITIES

Authorship is the assignment of ownership of a piece of written scholarship. Chapter 12 reviews the ethical considerations of authorship and provides guidelines for establishing author identification and order. At the time of submission, author identification and order should have been established. The first author, the author who has made the most substantial contributions to a study, is commonly but not always, the corresponding author. The corresponding author is the author who assumes responsibility for manuscript final preparation before submission, manuscript submission, all resubmissions, and all correspondence with the editor. It is the corresponding author's responsibility to ensure that the manuscript is prepared in accordance with author guidelines, that resubmissions thoroughly address requested revisions by editors and reviewers, that page proofs are correct and accurately reflect authors' work, and that copyright forms are correctly signed and submitted by all authors (or as required by a specific journal). Some journals provide the email address of the corresponding author so that researchers can contact this author about study content.

Gutman, S. A. *Journal Article Writing and Publication: Your Guide to Mastering Clinical Health Care Reporting Standards* (pp. 69-77). © 2017 Taylor & Francis Group.

Journal Selection

After authors have collected, analyzed, and interpreted data and are ready to write the manuscript narrative, they should begin to formulate ideas about the type of journals that best match their completed research. It is good practice to select two to three possible journals and rank each journal's congruence with your study. Most journals describe commonly published article types and publication goals in their author guidelines. Because dual or simultaneous submission to two or more journals is considered publication misconduct, authors should select one journal and use that journal's author guidelines to prepare and format their manuscript. Author guidelines can be easily located on a journal's website. Do not assume that you are familiar with a specific journal's author guidelines and fail to obtain them. Journals update author guidelines frequently, particularly as a result of changing copyright laws and new and revised reporting guidelines.

Following Author Guidelines and Formatting Styles

Once you have obtained the author guidelines for the journal to which you wish to submit, it is important to read the entire narrative and make notes about essential points, including the following:

- Page length requirements for the entire manuscript
- Word count requirements for the entire manuscript
- Spacing of type
- Font type and size
- Margin size
- Page numbering
- Abstract word count
- Abstract headings
- Use of key words
- Table and figure count limitations
- Requirements concerning permission to reprint published materials
- Masking procedures

Author guidelines will state which style guide should be used by authors to format manuscripts. In the health professions, many journals use the *Publication Manual of the American Psychological Association*, 6th ed. (American Psychological Association, 2010). Authors should obtain the indicated style guide and ensure that their manuscript adheres to style guide specifications; particular detailed attention should be paid to citation and reference formatting. Software programs are available that can convert references into a variety of style guide formats. Manuscripts that do not adhere to a journal's author guidelines and designated style guide format reflect poorly on a submission. Such manuscripts appear to have been previously submitted to and rejected by another journal. Manuscripts with numerous style guide and author guideline errors are more difficult for editors and reviewers to evaluate.

MANUSCRIPT MASKING

Most journals request that a masked manuscript be submitted alone or in addition to an unmasked copy. Masking means that all identifying author information (including names and affiliations) and institution names (i.e., the names of universities and clinical facilities) be removed from the manuscript. The acknowledgment section should also be removed from a masked manuscript copy. Using masked manuscripts in the review process enhances confidentiality and promotes ethical review processes. Commonly overlooked items that should be masked include the institutional review board's affiliated university name, the names of clinical facilities from which participants were recruited, and the authors' names in manuscript citations and references. Participant identities should never be revealed through manuscript photographs or by naming the clinical facility at which they received treatment.

WRITING CONCISELY AND PRECISELY

Many authors contact editors to justify why their papers should be published in excess of page length limitations. Such justifications usually address the significance of findings and the need to publish all results in one paper. There is never a defensible reason why a paper must be published in excess of page length requirements. If a paper is significantly over length, it should be revised into two separate papers. A paper that is moderately over length should be edited for conciseness. Authors should consider the following:

- Whether all tables/figures are essential or can be deleted or reduced in size
- Whether the literature addresses the focused topic or extends beyond material necessary to describe background information
- Whether the Discussion section is concise and conveys the simplest interpretation of findings or extends beyond study results

In many submissions, the Method section is not adequately described in accordance with transparent reporting standards and requires additional information. Key sections most commonly requiring editing to reduce length are the Introduction (and embedded literature review) and Discussion. Many manuscripts contain information in the Introduction and Discussion sections that is extraneous to the study presentation and can be removed. Authors must seek to write concisely and precisely—that is, formulate sentences conveying the greatest amount of meaning while using the least amount of words. Writing concisely and precisely is a learned skill that can be enhanced through writing practice, multiple paper revisions, and working with a competent editor who can edit papers for clarity, reduced length, and word choice precision. Such editors are commonly employed by authors for personal use; it is not the responsibility of journal editor-in-chiefs to assist with major manuscript editing. Writing concisely and precisely most clearly conveys the author's intended message to readers. The focused message of a manuscript should be described using simple language that is not lost in technical jargon and long discourses. Concise and precise language can be facilitated by the use of active voice. While traditional journal writing has encouraged authors to use third-person language, most journals now require authors to use active voice in an effort to enhance transparency of research procedures and researcher roles.

WRITING WITHOUT BIAS

Writing without bias involves presenting written ideas without prejudice or disposition regarding gender, sex, sexual orientation, race and ethnicity, disability, and age. Minimal reporting standards mandate that the participant demographics of sex, race/ethnicity, disability, and age should always be reported to promote transparency and reduce bias in research studies. This section provides guidance for authors to both identify and remove bias from written scholarship.

Gender, Sex, and Sexual Orientation

Gender is the cultural interpretation of male and female roles and is self-assigned based on the individual's personal feelings about being male or female in a particular social group (Rothenberg, 2013). Sex is the biological designation of male or female based on genetics and the appearance of reproductive organs. With gender reassignment surgery, mixed phenotype births (e.g., both male and female reproductive organs may be present), and a variety of chromosomal patterns (in which a phenotypic male may appear female and vice versa), sex assignment can be unclear and should be designated by study participants rather than researchers.

Sexual orientation is the self-identified attraction to males, females, or both (Conron, Mimiaga, & Landers, 2010) and should also be designated by participants rather than researchers. Unless your study specifically addresses sexual orientation as a variable that impacts results and data interpretation, sexual orientation should not be reported as a participant demographic. The reporting of sexual orientation when this demographic does not impact study findings is biased and implies that people with differing sexual orientations have innate differences from others beyond sexual attraction.

When reporting sex of participants, do not report one sex's *n* value without reporting the other's. For example, "There were 39 participants (male = 17)." Instead, report both: "There were 39 participants (male = 17; female = 22)." Reporting the number of only one group implies that the other group's data are unimportant.

Both sexes collectively should not be referred to as *mankind* or *man*; *humans* or *people* can be used instead. The pronoun *he* should not be used to refer to both sexes. For example, "A therapist can enhance his intervention fidelity by viewing videos of his practice sessions." Use plural pronouns instead: "Therapists can enhance their intervention fidelity by viewing videos of their practice sessions." Do not mix plural and singular pronouns in the same sentence: "A therapist can enhance their intervention fidelity by viewing videos of their clinical sessions." *A* is singular and *their* is plural, and they do not match grammatically. Avoid this commonly made mistake by ensuring that your pronouns in one sentence are either singular or plural but not both.

Race and Ethnicity

Race and ethnicity are essential in reporting standard demographics. *Race* is the classification of human groups based on specific genetic and biological markers. Race can also be based on national origin. *Ethnicity* is the classification of human groups based on cultural heritage. Race and ethnicity are based on participants' own identification, rather than the researchers'. When reporting race and ethnicity, use the preferred classification selected by participants. When constructing checklists for participants, use commonly accepted categories such as census categories and include "other" as an item with an option for participants to insert their own category. The reporting of race and ethnicity should be as specific as possible, such as Mexican American and Native American. Authors should report race and ethnicity using parallel terms, for example, African American and Asian American. Unparalleled terms in which one group is described by skin color and the other by cultural heritage (e.g., White and Pacific Islander) should be avoided. Racial and ethnic groups are considered to be proper nouns and should be capitalized: Black, White, Alaskan American.

Disability

When writing about participants with disability, it is important to use person-first language. Person-first language is a writing style in which the participant is not defined by the presence of disability. *Participants with schizophrenia* is an example of person-first writing. Conversely, *schizophrenic participants* inappropriately characterizes the participants by the presence of schizophrenia.

Similarly, language that qualifies the participants' experience through the researcher's lens is inappropriate. For example, *stroke victim, brain-damaged participants,* and "the participants suffered from multiple sclerosis" are examples in which the author has negatively labeled the participants' experience of disability.

The use of the word *normal* as a comparison to groups with disability is inappropriate. For example, it is inappropriate to use the following: "the normal control group," ". . . people with spinal cord injury compared to normal people in the population." The word *normal* when used to compare groups with and without disabilities implies that people having disabilities are abnormal or inferior to those without disabilities. Instead of *normal,* use *healthy control group, typically developed population,* and *typically developing children.*

Age

Participant ages and age ranges should always be provided as specifically as possible. Large, open-ended ranges such as *over 65* and *under 18* should be avoided. *Adolescents* refers to males and females aged 13 to 17 years, *preadolescents* refers to males and females aged 11 to 12 years, *children* refers to males and females aged 1 to 10 years, and *infants* refers to newborns to 11-month-olds. Males and females 18 years and older should be referred to as *adults.* The term *older adults* is preferred to the terms *seniors* and *elderly* (American Psychological Association, 2010).

Participants vs. Subjects

Traditionally the term *subjects* has been used in scientific journal writing in the hard sciences and in a time period before institutional review boards began to rigorously protect human participant and animal rights. In health care research, the term *participants* should be used instead of *subjects.* The term *subjects* implies that people may or may not know they are in a study and are being acted upon by the researcher. In health care writing, the term *participants* implies that people know they are part of a study and are actively participating.

SUBMISSION PROCESS

Most journals have online submission systems with specific instructions and fields that must be completed to successfully submit manuscripts. Prior to submission, authors must have formatted their manuscript in full accordance with the journal's author guidelines or the paper will likely be returned. Nonadherence to page length, abstract length, table/figure count, and masking instructions are common reasons why manuscripts are returned to authors.

Most journals require authors to confirm that the manuscript is original and is not being simultaneously submitted to another journal. While online submission systems commonly require the uploading of masked manuscripts, the system will ask that corresponding author and coauthor information (e.g., names, credentials, affiliations, and email addresses) be inserted in designated fields. It is important that such information be accurate and complete because this information commonly serves as the means through which editors and journal staff contact authors. If the corresponding author's contact information changes during the manuscript review process, it is essential to notify the editor and journal staff in writing immediately.

Many journals ask that authors either submit their own similar and derivative publications or notify editors of the existence of such work to prevent inadvertent copyright issues. Electronic plagiarism check software programs are commonly used by journals to identify possible copyright problems.

Journal online submission systems commonly allow authors to recommend specific reviewers whose expertise matches the manuscript subject matter. Similarly, journals often allow authors to identify reviewers who may be inappropriate for manuscript review because of conflicting interests.

Author guidelines usually provide parameters for manuscript review length. Online systems commonly have tracking systems through which authors can monitor the status of their manuscript review. It is not appropriate to contact the editor about manuscript review status until approximately 1 month after the review time period has expired. Reviewers frequently experience unanticipated life events that may delay the submission of paper reviews. Reviewers recommended by authors may have been difficult to secure, and the review process may have been delayed. Occasionally, reviewers diverge in their recommendations and an arbitrating reviewer must be secured who can provide a third opinion. The process of arbitration will extend the review process but will enhance its trustworthiness. If at any time during the submission and review process authors wish to withdraw their manuscript from consideration, they should contact the editor or journal staff immediately.

Checklist for Submission

- ☐ The corresponding author is identified, and contact information is provided (usually through the online system and not the manuscript).
- ☐ All coauthor information, including authorship order, has been accurately provided through the online system.
- ☐ The manuscript is fully masked.
- ☐ The manuscript formatting is congruent with the journal's designated style guidelines.
- ☐ All specific formatting guidelines that are unique to the journal and supersede the designated style guidelines have been adhered to.
- ☐ All citations in the text are referenced.
- ☐ All citations and references are congruent with regard to spelling and date.
- ☐ All tables and figures are referred to in the text and labeled in accordance with text order.
- ☐ All tables and figures have titles or captions.
- ☐ All permissions to reprint copyrighted material have been submitted.
- ☐ Supplemental materials that may be published online, but not in hard copy, are identified and submitted.

RESPONDING TO REVIEWER RECOMMENDATIONS

If you are invited to make revisions and resubmit your manuscript, congratulate yourself and thoroughly read all recommendations from the editor and reviewers. An invitation to revise and resubmit does not guarantee acceptance; it is important to understand requested recommendations, address revisions thoroughly, and submit a polished, higher quality revised manuscript.

The editor will likely specify instructions for responding to reviewer recommendations, but commonly authors should create a document in which all reviewer comments are listed and answered in writing. All responses to reviewer recommendations should be made in complete sentences and precisely describe how revisions address noted concerns. It is important to understand that this document will be read by both the original reviewers and editor to understand whether and how well the authors addressed noted concerns.

Responses to reviewer recommendations should be thorough and precise, as in the following examples:

Reviewer recommendation: In the Method section please insert a section, Interveners, in which you identify who provided intervention (type of professional), how many therapists provided intervention, their training for intervention administration, and whether interveners were blinded to group assignment.

Answer: In the Methods section, we inserted a section labeled "Interveners" and provided the following text on p. 11: "Two occupational therapists participated in intervention administration. Both possessed over 10 years of pediatric practice experience and were trained in intervention delivery by the first author. Training consisted of a 2-day seminar presented by the first and second authors. Both interveners were blinded to participant group assignment."

The following answers are inappropriate and do not provide sufficient information to help the reviewers and editor understand whether and how well the concern was addressed:

Answer: Done.

Answer: We added the information as requested.

Answer: This information can now be found on p. 11.

If authors do not agree with a particular reviewer recommendation, it is appropriate to write a response explaining why the revision was not needed. For example:

Reviewer recommendation: It would be helpful to discuss the work of Strauss in the literature review and relate it to the need for your study.

Answer: We appreciate the recommendation to address Strauss' work in our literature review; however, because Strauss' work specifically addresses hemiplegia and our intervention addresses anosognosia, and because of page limitations, we decided to forgo this recommendation. Instead, we briefly discussed how Strauss' findings support our own in the Discussion section.

Most reviews are written professionally and offer constructive guidance to authors. Occasionally, reviewers inappropriately allow their emotions to permeate the language of a written review. As a result, the review language may be harsh or negative. When this occurs, authors should not personalize the tone of the review but instead focus only on the recommendations and maintain professional, neutral language in their written responses to the reviewers and editor. Maintaining professionalism includes thanking the editor and reviewers for their feedback and the opportunity to revise the manuscript.

Similarly, journal reviewers should thank authors for the opportunity to review their manuscript and adopt positive, emotionally neutral language in written reviews. All reviews should be written constructively and help authors understand how to strengthen their manuscripts. Even reviews that recommend rejection should be written positively and help authors understand how their study could be enhanced if conducted in the future.

Once authors have made requested revisions and created their "response to reviewer comments" document, the manuscript can then be resubmitted in accordance with journal guidelines. Editors commonly provide resubmission deadlines, which should be adhered to as closely as possible. If authors cannot resubmit their manuscript by a specified deadline, the corresponding author should contact the editor to request an extension. Once resubmitted, the revised manuscript will likely be reviewed by one or both of the original reviewers to determine whether the manuscript now meets publication standards. Further revisions may be requested. The manuscript revision and resubmission process is a lengthy one but provides the opportunity for authors to enhance their writing skills and become concise, precise writers.

Revising and Submitting to Another Journal if Rejected

If you receive a rejection letter from a journal, do not become discouraged. Go to the next journal on your list and determine whether that journal's publication goals match your work. Remember that journals are only able to publish a limited amount of articles, have specific publication goals, and may only publish articles about a limited topic range. Approximately 50% of rejected manuscripts are not well suited to the journal to which they were submitted. Make sure that your work matches well with the next journal to which you submit.

Go through the editor's and reviewers' comments to understand why your paper was rejected from the first journal. Make a list of noted concerns and address these as thoroughly as possible in the manuscript's next revision. Ask a neutral colleague to read your revised manuscript and provide feedback. Obtain the author guidelines from your next selected journal and reformat your manuscript to match the specified style guidelines.

The submission and publication process is lengthy and involves multiple drafts, revisions, and possible rejections. Understanding this process, learning how to refrain from personalizing feedback and rejection, and making the time commitment for writing will help you to hurdle setbacks and rejections and persevere to eventual publication. The more frequently you go through this process, the easier it becomes.

Checklist for Preparing and Submitting Manuscripts for Publication

- ☐ Before submission, establish author order and designate the corresponding author.
- ☐ Select two to three journals whose publication goals match your study or paper topic.
- ☐ Obtain the author guidelines of each journal to determine publication goals.
- ☐ Rank the order of journals in accordance with congruence with your work.
- ☐ Select one journal and follow that journal's style guidelines and formatting instructions.
- ☐ Make sure that the manuscript does not exceed journal page length and word count requirements.
- ☐ Work with a professional editor or neutral colleague who can proof the manuscript for concise, precise grammatical structure and sentence meaning.
- ☐ Make sure that the writing is not biased with regard to gender, sex, race and ethnicity, disability, and age.
- ☐ Use the term *participants* rather than *subjects* throughout the manuscript.
- ☐ Before submission, prepare a fully masked manuscript.
- ☐ In the submission process, indicate that the manuscript is original and is not being simultaneously submitted to another journal.

- ☐ Provide corresponding author and coauthor information fully and accurately.
- ☐ Submit or disclose to the editor any similar or derivative publications to prevent inadvertent copyright issues.
- ☐ If requested, provide the editor with names of recommended reviewers and reviewers having conflicting interests.
- ☐ If available, use the online tracking system to monitor your manuscript's status in the review process. Contact the editor only if you have not received information by 1 month after the allotted review period has ended.
- ☐ Contact the editor if you wish to withdraw the manuscript from review.
- ☐ If invited to revise your manuscript, address all editor and reviewer comments thoroughly.
- ☐ Prepare a document in which all editor and reviewer comments are listed followed by thorough and precise answers.
- ☐ Maintain neutral and professional language and tone in all contact with editors and reviewers. Thank reviewers and editors for their feedback and the opportunity to revise and resubmit.
- ☐ If rejected, go to the next journal on your list and follow the author guidelines to reformat your manuscript.
- ☐ Use the first journal's reviewer comments to revise the manuscript as much as possible.
- ☐ Submit to the next journal.

REFERENCES

American Psychological Association. (2010). *Publication manual of the American Psychological Association* (6th ed.). Washington, DC: Author.

Conron, K. J., Mimiaga, M. J., & Landers, S. J. (2010). A population-based study of sexual orientation identity and gender differences in adult health. *American Journal of Public Health, 100*(10), 1953–1960. doi:10.2105/AJPH.2009.174169

Rothenberg, P. S. (2013). *Race, class, and gender in the United States: An integrated study* (9th ed.). New York, NY: Worth.

9

The Revision Process

The process of writing and submitting a paper to a scholarly journal involves revision in which reviewers and editors provide feedback and recommendations to enhance a manuscript's publication readiness. All manuscripts—even those written by seasoned scholars—go through the revision process. As authors, we may have already revised papers through multiple drafts before submission. Revisions requested by journal reviewers and editors may feel extraneous after revisions that authors have made prior to submission. However, journal reviewer recommendations are important because they emerge through the lens of professionals who best understand the publication requirements and objectives of a particular journal to which the paper was submitted.

As authors we may become attached to our writing and feel resistant to revision requests. Such attachment often hinders our ability to understand how papers can be improved. It is important to remember that all published articles have gone through moderate to extensive revisions after initial journal submission. Even after paper acceptance, copyeditors will likely further edit papers to enhance clarity and reduce word length. These steps are important components of the revision process and, while difficult to experience emotionally, ultimately enhance an article's final presentation.

DEPERSONALIZING REVIEWER FEEDBACK

Reviewer feedback can feel critical even when it was not intended to be. It is important to set aside emotions when receiving reviewer feedback to best understand how requested revisions can strengthen a manuscript. To depersonalize reviewer comments, it is important that authors view their paper as a draft that will be revised and strengthened multiple times. After initially reading reviewer feedback, it is often beneficial to set the manuscript aside for a day or more before making revisions. This time may help authors to reduce initial emotional reactions to reviewer feedback and begin to perceive how requested revisions can be incorporated.

Gutman, S. A. *Journal Article Writing and Publication: Your Guide to Mastering Clinical Health Care Reporting Standards* (pp. 79-126). © 2017 Taylor & Francis Group.

Occasionally, reviewer comments can be harsh and unprofessional. Reviews should not be written in emotionally laden language or negative comments. Editors are responsible for flagging unprofessionally written reviews and addressing them before they are provided to authors. Unfortunately, unprofessionally written reviews are not always modified before reaching authors. When authors receive such reviews, they must separate themselves emotionally from the review language and concentrate on the feedback that can be used to strengthen their manuscript.

It is important that authors do not become so daunted by reviewer feedback that they postpone making revisions and allow a paper to die. Publication requires perseverance and a thick skin able to withstand critique. The more authors experience the journal writing and submission process, the easier it becomes.

UNDERSTANDING REVIEW FEEDBACK

After separating authors' emotions from the review process—so that emotions do not influence the ability to understand reviewer feedback—authors should reread all comments and begin to generate ideas for incorporating requested revisions into the next draft. It is important at this stage that authors fully understand what reviewers have requested. If authors are uncertain regarding the meaning of reviewer feedback for a specific item, they should first consult with coauthors and colleagues. The editor should be contacted directly if a specific reviewer comment cannot be interpreted.

Once they understand all comments, authors should identify those revisions that will be addressed and generate ideas about how revisions will be made. Occasionally, reviewers request revisions that authors believe to be inappropriate. It is suitable for authors to refrain from making a specific requested revision when such a revision may move the paper in an unintended direction or add significant word length that is incongruent with journal guidelines. In this case, authors should justify their decision in writing to the editor and reviewers (as discussed later in this chapter).

Editors often specify due dates by which revisions should be resubmitted, and such due dates should be adhered to as closely as possible. When authors cannot resubmit by a specific due date, they should request a written extension from the editor. Certain types of revisions will require greater time and effort than others. For example, updating references, reducing word count, and adding minor detail are revisions that can be made relatively quickly. Most papers require reducing detail in the Introduction section, inserting additional clarifying information in the Method section, and elaborating on interpretive information provided in the Discussion section. These types of revisions require greater time and labor. Revisions requiring statistical reanalysis, reorganization of content, substantial addition of information, and reinterpretation of results are the most labor intensive and require a comprehensive overhaul. It is essential to correctly estimate the time needed for revisions, develop a timeline, and adhere to it so that the manuscript can be resubmitted by the appointed due date. Manuscripts that are not resubmitted by the appointed due date and have not received an extension from the editor will often be withdrawn by a journal.

ADHERING TO WORD LIMITS

During the revision process, it is critical to adhere to the journal's specified word and page counts. Many authors who are asked to insert background, clarifying, and interpretative information make the mistake of adding content without adjusting other manuscript sections to adhere to the journal's word limit. Revisions that exceed the maximum length by several hundred words are often resubmitted without thought to word count specifications. This oversight prolongs the revision process because the paper must be revised again to reduce word count. Before authors begin revisions, they should recheck journal guidelines regarding word count and reread the editor's cover letter to determine whether they must maintain this limit or are permitted to exceed it by a circumscribed amount. If in doubt, authors should contact the editor about word count limitations.

RESPONDING TO REVIEWER COMMENTS

Editors commonly provide instructions to authors indicating how responses to reviewer comments should be made. In addition to making requested revisions directly in the manuscript text, most journals request that authors generate a separate document in which they list all reviewer comments followed by author responses (see pages 101-106). Editors and reviewers will consult this document to understand how authors addressed each requested revision item. Authors should not take a casual approach to making these responses. All author responses should be made in complete, clear sentences that directly answer reviewer questions and concerns.

Example of Appropriate Response to Reviewers

Reviewer comment: In the Data Analysis section of the Methods, please specify which statistical test was used to determine whether differences between treatment and control groups existed at baseline. Please provide a citation for this test.

Author response: In the Data Analysis section of the Methods, we inserted the following sentence: "A Wilcoxon signed-rank test was used to determine whether a statistically significant difference existed between treatment and control groups on pretest scores (Portney & Watkins, 2008)."

Example of Inappropriate Responses to Reviewers

Author response: Done.
Author response: We added this information.
Author response: This information is now added at line 113.

JUSTIFYING OMISSION OF REQUESTED REVISIONS

Occasionally, reviewers request revisions that are incongruent with the authors' study objectives and intent. Authors do not need to make all requested revisions if they are able to justify why a specific requested revision is unsuitable. Such justifications should be made in the document listing responses to reviewer comments.

Example

Reviewer comment: Please include information about transactional theory in the introduction and relate this information to the theoretical basis for your intervention.

Author response: Thank you for this suggestion. Although we agree that transactional theory could be viewed as a basis for our intervention, we did not use this theory in our intervention development process. As noted in the Introduction, we instead used Prochaska and DiClemente's stages of change model (transtheoretical theory) as a basis for our intervention. Because of manuscript length limitations, and because of additional requested content that further added page length, we chose not to address an additional theoretical base in the Introduction. We will, however, defer to the editor regarding this decision.

In the previous author response, the authors address the recommendation by thanking the reviewer for the suggestion and using appropriate language to explain why an additional theoretical base would be redundant. The authors do not suggest that the recommendation is unsuitable. Rather they use neutral language to explain that an additional theory description would add word length that would cause the paper to exceed specified limitations. They appropriately end their response by stating that they will make this revision if desired by the editor.

Although reviewer recommendations can be challenged by authors, authors should generally comply with editor instructions—particularly when instructions address such things as word count length, formatting requirements, style guide use, heading use, and compliance with standard research reporting guidelines. Failure to defer to the above types of editor directions can result in paper rejection. Authors should not petition editors for permission to extend manuscript page length or table and figure counts.

Etiquette of the Review Process

The review process has its own set of etiquette rules that govern author, editor, and reviewer roles and behaviors. All parties should maintain neutral, positive language in all correspondence. Before the advent of email, when journal correspondence was carried out through mailed letters, correspondence adhered to widely accepted rules for professional behavior and language. Email and the breakdown of our society's social formality have loosened rules for journal correspondence. Too often, the instantaneous communication of email has encouraged people to send inappropriate, unprofessional correspondence in immediate reaction, without thinking about consequences. I urge authors to send well-considered correspondence after sufficiently processing emotional reactions in response to the review process. I also recommend the following guidelines for correspondence:

- Authors should not send correspondence when they have an emotional response to the review process. It is beneficial to wait several days to process emotions before sending correspondence.

- All correspondence should use positive language. Even if authors believe that they received an unprofessional review with emotionally laden language, it is essential not to respond similarly.

- All language in the document listing responses to reviewer comments should be neutral and positive, even if authors believe that the reviewer was unprofessional.

- To maintain professionalism, authors should thank the editor and reviewers for their help in all correspondence, particularly in their responses to reviewer comments.

- Authors should use the journal's online tracking system to determine the status of their manuscript review. Authors should not contact the editor until 1 month has expired beyond the allotted review time. A journal's author guidelines will usually specify the average review length; however, reviewer crises and difficulty securing appropriate reviewers for a specific topic can slow the average review process.

- Authors should not contact the journal to persuade the editor to review the manuscript faster to accommodate author needs (e.g., publications needed to apply for promotion or tenure or a desire to have articles published in the same issue).

- Authors should expect at least two manuscript revisions and resubmissions before acceptance.

- Authors should understand that manuscript revision does not guarantee acceptance. On occasion, authors are not able to make revisions in accordance with journal standards despite considerable help from editors and reviewers.

PROOFREAD PRIOR TO RESUBMISSION

After requested revisions have been completed and prior to journal resubmission, authors should thoroughly proof the revised manuscript to identify and correct grammatical and stylistic errors, inconsistencies between citations and references, and inconsistencies between text and tables. Table numbers and heading levels can be mislabeled and lose organization through multiple paper drafts. Such problems commonly occur inadvertently during manuscript revisions. When unidentified and uncorrected, such errors can make a manuscript appear sloppily and hastily revised and further prolong the review process. On occasion authors become so familiar with a manuscript that they no longer easily see errors. In such cases, it is beneficial to have a coauthor or colleague proof the text before resubmission.

EXAMPLE OF A MANUSCRIPT REVISION PROCESS

To illustrate how a submitted manuscript is revised based on reviewer feedback, I present the initial and revised drafts of the article *Development and Psychometric Properties of the Emotional Intelligence Admission Essay Scale* (Gutman & Falk-Kessler, 2016). Reviewer comments and author responses are also included. This article was published in the 2016 summer issue of the *Open Journal of Occupational Therapy*, which is an open-access journal in which authors retain copyright. Reviewer comments are provided with permission of the journal's editor in chief.

Running head: EMOTIONAL INTELLIGENCE ADMISSION ESSAY SCALE

Development and Psychometric Properties of the

Emotional Intelligence Admission Essay Scale

Sharon A. Gutman, PhD, OTR, FAOTA

Janet P. Falk-Kessler, EdD, OTR, FAOTA

Abstract

Objective: The purpose was to describe the development and psychometric properties of the Emotional

Intelligence Admission Essay scale.

Methods: The authors developed an admission essay question and rating scale designed to provide

information about applicants' emotional intelligence (EI). Content validity, convergent validity, inter-

rater reliability, and internal consistency were established. The scale was also examined to determine

if it could discriminate between students with and without professional behavior problems in the aca-

demic and fieldwork settings.

Results: Content validity was found to be high by a panel of three experts in EI (content validity

index = 1.0). Convergent validity with the Assessing Emotions Scale was moderate ($r = .46, p < .02$).

Interrater reliability between two trained faculty raters was high ($ICC = .91, p < .000$). Internal con-

sistency of the scale was high with a Cronbach's alpha of .95. This version of the scale was not able to

discriminate between students with and without professional behavior problems.

Conclusion: The moderate to strong psychometric properties suggest that the EI Admission Essay

Scale has the ability to provide information about applicants' EI. The wording of the essay question

must be modified to better instruct applicants to address interpersonal conflict.

Keywords: occupational therapy, admission selection, instrument development

Emotional intelligence (EI) is a form of social intelligence that involves the ability to recognize and appraise emotions in oneself and others, regulate and manage emotions in oneself and others, and use emotion based information to guide behavior and problem solving (Arora et al., 2010). The term was first developed by Salovey and Mayer (1990) who argued that EI was a distinct set of skills that were separate from personality traits and previously identified types of intelligence. Later researchers extended the definition of EI by dissecting the construct into inter- and intrapersonal intelligences wherein interpersonal intelligence involves the ability to accurately read and assess other's verbal and nonverbal expressions; easily build rapport with others using an open, compassionate countenance that demonstrates interest in others; and successfully diffuse and negotiate interpersonal conflict (Carrothers, Gregory, & Gallagher, 2000; McQueen, 2004). Intrapersonal intelligence involves the ability to recognize emotion in oneself and understand its origin, be aware of how one's emotions impact one's behaviors and influence others, and monitor and regulate one's emotions to enhance emotional stability and wellness (Elam, 2000; McQueen, 2004).

Emotional intelligence is a critical skill for occupational therapists and clinical competencies relating to EI involve the ability to collaboratively work with a team of health care professionals; identify and manage patient emotions to adeptly address patient concerns and needs; identify and manage team member emotions to promote patient advocacy and diffuse possible professional domain conflicts; communicate with patients, family members, caregivers, health care providers, and insurers to ensure optimal patient care; educate caregivers who may feel overwhelmed and ill-prepared to assume caregiving responsibilities; and work cooperatively and compassionately with people from varied and diverse cultural groups (McQueen, 2004; Victoroff & Boyatzis, 2013). Given the great extent of clinical competencies that directly relate to emotional intelligence, it is surprising that this construct has not been formally examined in occupational therapy admission selection criteria.

Occupational therapy program admission selection criteria have traditionally relied upon the cognitive measures of cumulative grade point average (GPA), prerequisite GPA, science GPA, and preadmission standardized tests such as the Graduate Record Exam (GRE) (Romanelli, Cain, & Smith, 2006). Traditionally used noncognitive measures have included interviews, personal statements and essays, volunteerism, and prior service and healthcare experience (Jones-Schenk & Harper, 2014). While the above cognitive and noncognitive measures have been shown to provide accurate predictive information about an applicant's academic performance in graduate school (Carr, 2009), they do not provide information about an applicant's potential clinical performance and professional behaviors in the academic program and fieldwork experiences. Given the large number of occupational therapy clinical competencies that relate to EI, it seems prudent to have an admission criterion that measures an applicant's EI and can identify students who have both the academic skill and EI needed to succeed in an occupational therapy program and career. The need for an EI measure in the admission selection process has been elevated by the growing number of occupational therapy school applications in the last decades (American Occupational Therapy Association [AOTA], 2014), the inflation of academic grades at the college and university level lessening the rigor of GPA as a reliable assessment measure (Jewell, McPherson, & Tieslau, 2013), and the generational difference in students applying to health care programs who may have values and professional behaviors that are incongruent with health care professions and who may be qualitatively different from applicants of past decades (Romanelli et al., 2006).

Other health care professions have begun to recognize the value of using EI measures in the admission selection process. Much of the literature addressing the EI of health care student applicants has been generated by the professions of medicine, nursing, dentistry, and pharmacy (Arora, et al., 2010; Lyon, Trotter, Holt, Powell, & Roe 2013; Romanelli et al., 2006; Victoroff & Boyatzis, 2013). These studies have found that students with high levels of EI as measured on standardized assessments demonstrate higher levels of clinical performance (Codier, Kofoed, & Peters, 2015; Hannah, Lim, & Ayers, 2009; Rankin, 2013), are more highly rated by clinical supervisors and patients (Arora et al., 2010; Hannah et al., 2009; Rankin, 2013; Victoroff & Boyatzis, 2013), are more likely to complete their professional health care education programs (Jones-Schenk & Harper, 2014; Rankin, 2013), and are better able to work collaboratively on treatment teams as assessed by supervisors (Arora et al., 2010; Victoroff & Boyatzis, 2013). Most of the EI measures used in these studies were administered to students already matriculated in health care programs and all authors supported the need for the incorporation of EI measures administered during the admission process.

Although the need for and value of EI measures used during the admission selection process of health care programs is clear, the most practical and reliable type of EI measure is of debate. The most commonly available form of EI measure is a paper and pencil or computer generated test (Arora et al., 2010). Such assessments either pose scenarios and ask respondents to identify the most emotionally intelligent answer through a multiple choice format or are self-report measures that ask respondents to identify to what extent they identify with a specific skill (e.g., "I am able to read other's facial expressions to determine their mood.") (Fiori & Antonakis, 2011). Another form of EI assessment gaining interest among health care programs is the structured interview, in which a specific set of questions is asked of all applicants (Latif, 2004; Levashina, Hartwell, Morgeson, & Campion, 2014; Pau et al., 2013). In the structured interview, applicants may be consecutively interviewed by several interviewers who are all trained in interview administration and have established interrater reliability in the use of a standardized EI rating scale. While the use of face-to-face structured interviews and standardized paper and pencil or computer generated tests are often reliable and valid, they can be costly and labor intensive. Most EI measures with established reliability and validity are expensive and an administration fee is charged per student. Structured interviewing is time and labor intensive and requires training interviewers in both administration and assessment.

In response to the need to incorporate a practical and reliable EI measure into the admission selection process, the faculty in the Occupational Therapy Program at Columbia University Medical Center (CUMC), have developed an essay question and rating scale, the EI Admission Essay Scale, which may have the ability to provide information about an applicant's EI. The essay question asks applicants to describe a conflict situation in a work, school, or personal event; how the applicant knowingly or unknowingly contributed to the conflict; and how he or she attempted to resolve the conflict based on the ability to use emotion based information to guide problem solving. The instrument used to assess the applicant's essay is a 5-item, 4-point Likert scale with a range from 0 (no evidence) to 3 (strong evidence). The purpose of the present study was to develop the pilot version of the EI Admission Essay Scale, and establish content and convergent validity, interrater reliability, and internal consistency. Additionally, we hoped to determine whether the scale is able to discriminate between students who have professional behavior problems in the academic and fieldwork setting and students who do not.

The research questions were:

1. Can an admission essay question and rating scale be developed to provide information about an applicant's EI?

2. Using a panel of three experts in emotional intelligence research, what is the content validity of the EI Admission Essay Scale?

3. Does the EI Admission Essay Scale have convergent validity with the Assessing Emotions Scale (Schutte et al., 1998; Schutte, Malouff, & Bhullar, 2009)?

4. Using trained occupational therapy faculty raters, can interrater reliability be established for the EI Admission Essay Scale?

5. What is the internal consistency of the EI Admission Essay Scale using data from first year students in the CUMC Occupational Therapy Entry-Level Program?

6. Can the EI Admission Essay Scale discriminate between students who have professional behavior problems in the academic and/or fieldwork setting and students who do not?

Method

Research Design

This study described the development of a pilot assessment intended to measure EI in occupational therapy program applicants. Psychometric properties of the pilot instrument that were established included content and convergent validity, interrater reliability, and internal consistency as described below. We additionally examined whether the EI Admission Essay Scale could discriminate between students with and without professional behavior problems. CUMC's IRB approved this study and all participants provided consent.

Phase 1: Content Validity

Participants. To establish content validity of the EI Admission Essay Scale we assembled a panel of three professionals having expertise in EI research and literature. One expert was a physician educator who developed and implemented admission interview procedures for medical school applicants to ascertain information about EI. A second expert was a director of student wellness at a large, urban, northeastern university and specialized in emotional intelligence. A third expert was a professor in the Center for Educational Research and Evaluation at CUMC and taught coursework in EI.

Procedures. To develop the essay question and rating scale, the authors completed a literature review of emotional intelligence research and divided the construct into its component parts of intra- and interpersonal intelligence. Since successful conflict negotiation is a key determinant of higher levels of emotional intelligence, we developed a question in which applicants were asked to describe a conflict situation that occurred in a work, school, or personal situation. To gain insight into the applicant's awareness of ways in which his or her behavior and emotions impacted others (intrapersonal intelligence), applicants were asked to describe how they may have knowingly or unknowingly contributed to the conflict. To gain information about the applicant's ability to consider others' emotions and work collaboratively (interpersonal intelligence), we then asked applicants to describe their attempts at conflict resolution. Applicants were asked to address this question in 750 words. The question read as follows: "Describe a conflict that existed in a class, job, or life event in which you were a participant. How did you contribute wittingly or unwittingly to this conflict? How was the conflict handled by all involved parties?"

To develop a rating scale that could evaluate the EI content of the essay, we returned to our list of component parts of EI and formulated five scale items that addressed both intra- and interpersonal intelligence as described next. The scale items more heavily focus on interpersonal skills since such skills underlie a majority of clinical professional behaviors.

1. The applicant was able to place self in others' shoes to understand others' experiences, emotions, and perspectives in a conflict situation. (Interpersonal intelligence)

2. The applicant was able to understand how one's own actions contributed to a conflict. (Intrapersonal intelligence)

3. The applicant attempted to understand the conflict situation without blaming others for the conflict. (Interpersonal intelligence)

4. The applicant attempted to create a resolution that benefited all parties of a conflict to the greatest extent possible. (Interpersonal intelligence)

5. The applicant was able to cooperate equally with others in a conflict situation to problem solve and form a resolution to the conflict (i.e., did not monopolize problem solving or present oneself as hero). (Interpersonal intelligence)

Data collection. Expert raters were then provided with the essay question, list of scale items, and a rating scale form and were asked to complete and return the rating form via email. Experts did not consult with one another or have access to each other's scores.

Data analysis. We then completed a content validity ratio (CVR) (Lawshe, 1975) by asking the three experts to determine whether each scale item was congruent with the construct of EI. Experts rated each scale item using a three-point scale where 0 = not essential, 1 = useful, and 2 = essential. The CVR for each item was calculated using the formula below where ne is the number of experts who rated the item as essential and N is the total number of experts.

$$CVR = \frac{ne - N/2}{N/2}$$

A content validity index (CVI), the score for the entire instrument, was then calculated by determining the mean for all retained items (Lawshe suggests that items receiving a 0 be discarded). Using a content validity index, items require a .83 level of endorsement to establish content validity (DeVon et al., 2007); however, if 4 or fewer raters are used, the CVR for each item must be 1 to demonstrate content validity.

After content validity was established for the five scale items, we developed a 4-point rating scale for all items where 0 = no evidence, 1 = minimal evidence, 2 = moderate evidence, and 3 = strong evidence. Possible total scores range from 0 to 15 with higher scores indicating higher EI.

Results. All three experts rated each of the five essay scale items as essential (2.0) which resulted in a CVR of 1.0 for each item and a CVI of 1.0 for the entire scale. As a result, this pilot version of the scale was determined to have high content validity with the construct of EI.

Phase 2: Convergent Validity

Participants. To enroll in this study participants had to be matriculated first or second year students in the CUMC Occupational Therapy Entry-Level Program who completed the EI Admission Essay Scale as part of their application process. Participation was voluntary and students could choose not to participate. Students were recruited through an email invitation with an embedded link to an online version of the Assessing Emotions Scale (Schutte et al., 1998, 2009). We retrospectively collected admission essay questions of applicants enrolled as current first and second year students.

Procedures. To establish convergent validity we correlated EI Admission Essay Scale scores of 40 first and second year students with their scores on the Assessing Emotions Scale (Schutte et al., 1998, 2009). The Assessing Emotions Scale is a self-report measure of EI based on Salovey and Mayer's (1990) original model of EI (Mayer & Salovey, 1993). The scale has 33 items, uses a 5-point scale (1 = strongly disagree, 2 = somewhat disagree, 3 = neither agree nor disagree, 4 = somewhat agree, 5 = strongly agree), and requires approximately 5 minutes to complete. Total scores range from 33 to 165 with higher scores indicating higher levels of EI. Internal consistency of the scale was reported to be high with a Cronbach's alpha of .90 (Schutte et al., 1998, 2009). Schutte also reported that test-retest reliability was moderately high ($r = .78, p < .05$). Convergent validity with the Emotional Quotient Inventory (Bar-On, 1997) was found to be moderate ($r = .43, p < .05$) (Schutte et al., 1998, 2009).

Data collection. Both first and second year participating students completed the Assessing Emotions Scale during the same 1-month period; however, first year students completed the scale in the first semester of their academic program, while second year students completed the scale in the third semester of their academic program. To determine that length in the academic program did not influence student EI scores, we analyzed whether a statistically significant difference existed between first and second year student scores on both the EI Admission Essay Scale and the Assessing Emotions Scale.

The essay questions, which had been completed as part of the application process, were retrieved from student files by an admissions coordinator who coded and masked them. Students completed the Assessing Emotions Scale anonymously using their university ID numbers as codes. The master list linking codes to student names was maintained electronically on a password protected and encrypted computer by the admissions coordinator.

Both authors rated all 40 student EI Admission Essay Scales, first separately and then together to establish consensus when disagreement occurred. All essays were masked and authors were blinded to each other's initial scores. Interrater reliability between both authors was found to be high for separate, blinded ratings ($ICC = .94, p < .01$).

Data analysis. Data were entered into SPSS version 21 and level of significance was set at .05. To determine if EI Admission Essay Scale scores correlated with scores of the Assessing Emotions Scale, a Spearman rho correlation coefficient was used (Portney & Watkins, 2013).

Results. The data from 27 first year and 13 second year students (N = 40; male = 7, female = 33; White = 31, Asian = 5, African American = 2, Native American = 1, Hispanic = 1) were used to establish convergent validity between the EI Admission Essay Scale and the Assessing Emotions Scale. Convergent validity between these two scales was found to be moderate at $r = .46, p < .02$. Because first and second year students completed the Assessing Emotions Scale at different times in their curricula, we used a Mann Whitney U test to examine whether first and second year students differed in their EI levels (Portney & Watkins, 2013). A difference found may have been attributed to year in program; however, no statistically significant difference was found between first and second year students on both their EI Admission Essay Scale scores and the Assessing Emotions Scale scores.

Phase 3: Interrater Reliability

Participants. To establish interrater reliability of the EI Admission Essay Scale, two faculty members of the CUMC Occupational Therapy Program volunteered to serve as raters. These faculty members responded to an email invitation sent by the first author to all 10 full-time faculty members of the CUMC Occupational Therapy Program.

Procedures. The two faculty members received one hour of training in EI Admission Essay Scale rating procedures; training was provided by the first author. After training, raters were asked to separately rate three masked essays randomly selected from the total pool of 54 essays submitted by the first year class; essays were randomly selected by authors using a table of random numbers.

Data collection. The raters' scores for the three essays were completed separately and submitted by email one day after their training period. Raters were blinded to each other's scores.

Data analysis. Data were entered into SPSS version 21 and level of significance was set at .05. An intraclass correlation coefficient was used to determine interrater reliability between the two trained raters (Portney & Watkins, 2013).

Results. Interrater reliability was found to be high (*ICC* = .91, $p < .000$).

Phase 4: Internal Consistency

Participants. To determine the internal consistency of the EI Admission Essay Scale, we used the retrospectively collected admission essays of the 54 applicants admitted as current first year students (male = 10, female = 44; White = 44, Asian = 4, African American = 4, two or more races = 3).

Procedures. The essays of the 54 matriculated first year students were retrieved by the admissions coordinator who masked and coded them. Authors had already rated all essays during the procedures used to establish convergent validity. As stated above, essays were rated by both authors, first separately while blinded to each other's scores, and then together to address the existence of differences until consensus was reached. Achieving consensus was important to create one score for each essay item so that internal consistency could be determined. Interrater reliability between both authors for blinded rating was high ($ICC = .94$, $p < .01$). After the essays of all 54 first year students were rated by both authors and one score was established for each item (for all essays), the item scores for all essays were compared to determine internal consistency.

Data collection. Students completed the EI essays approximately 6 to 8 months earlier as part of their admissions application. This data set was retrospectively collected for this study by the admissions coordinator. Essays were masked and authors were blinded to each other's scores in the initial phase of rating.

Data analysis. Data were entered into SPSS version 21 and level of significance was set at .05. To determine if a correlation existed between scale items, a Cronbach's alpha correlation coefficient was used (Portney & Watkins, 2013).

Results. Internal consistency was found to be high with a Cronbach's alpha of .95.

Phase 5: Discrimination between Problematic and Nonproblematic Students

Participants. Data were the retrospectively collected admission essays of 54 admitted first year students.

Procedures. One objective of this study was to determine if the EI Admission Essay Scale could discriminate between students who demonstrated professional behavior problems in the academic and fieldwork environments and those who did not. We decided not to determine if EI Admission Essay Scale scores correlated with student scores on the American Occupational Therapy Association (AOTA) Fieldwork Evaluation (AOTA, 2002) because raters of the AOTA assessment had not attained interrater reliability with each other. Instead we first identified those students who demonstrated problematic professional behaviors in the academic and fieldwork environments and then determined if a statistically significant difference existed between their EI Admission Essay Scale scores and the scores of students who did not demonstrate professional behavior problems. Students who were identified as having problematic professional behaviors in the academic setting had received professional development forms and counseling from advisors. Students identified as exhibiting problematic professional behaviors in the fieldwork setting (Level I or II) had received behavioral contracts or had been withdrawn from or failed fieldwork.

Data collection. Data used to determine whether EI Admission Essay Scale scores could discriminate between problematic and nonproblematic students were the student EI Admission Essay Scale scores, student records of professional development forms (indicating that the student was counseled by the academic advisor as a result of problematic professional behaviors), and documentation of fieldwork behavioral contracts or withdrawal/failure. Examining whether the EI Admission Essay Scale could discriminate between students with and without professional behavior problems required that we unmask and link essays with academic and fieldwork performance information. For this reason, we completed this step as a final study activity to avoid biasing the procedures used to establish convergent validity, interrater reliability, and internal consistency.

Data analysis. To determine if the EI Admission Essay Scale could discriminate between students who experienced professional behavior problems and those who did not, we used a Mann Whitney U test (Portney & Watkins, 2013).

Results. Five students (male = 2; female = 3) demonstrated problematic professional behavior in the academic and fieldwork settings during the first year curriculum. A Mann Whitney U test showed no statistically significant difference between the EI Admission Essay Scale scores of these 5 students and the remaining 49 of the first year class. Despite a lack of statistical significance, however, it is interesting to note that these five students all obtained scores of 0 on their EI Admission Essay Scales, indicating the lowest possible score. Other students, however, also obtained 0 scores because they either failed to answer the question or showed no evidence of EI in their essays. When examining the 54 essays as a whole we found that only 18 (33.33%) answered the question and wrote about an experience of interpersonal conflict. Sixteen (29.62%) misinterpreted the question and wrote about an internal conflict that did not involve the ability to interpret and address others' emotions; 20 (37.03%) did not answer the question and wrote about their background, achievements, and career goals. Because of the large number of students who did not adequately answer the question and received low or 0 scores, it was difficult to statistically discriminate between students who possessed professional behavior problems and those who did not.

Discussion

This study aimed to determine if an admission essay scale could be developed that could capture information about an applicant's EI. The study also sought to establish the psychometric properties of content validity, convergent validity, interrater reliability, and internal consistency for this pilot version of the EI Admission Essay Scale. Because high content validity was established with a panel of experts and moderate convergent validity was found between the EI Admission Essay Scale and the Assessing Emotions Scale, we suggest that the EI Admission Essay Scale can yield information about an applicant's EI.

Although we hoped that the EI Admission Essay Scale could discriminate between students with and without professional behavior problems, we found that this version of the essay question was not able to do so, primarily because a large number of student applicants misinterpreted the question and wrote about an internal conflict rather than an interpersonal one. Although student essays addressing internal conflicts did provide some information about EI, essay content failed to address information about interpersonal intelligence. We realize that our question must be rewritten to provide clearer instructions about required essay content, particularly addressing interpersonal conflict. Once the question is rewritten we believe that the essay will have greater potential to yield information about EI and possibly predictive validity with classroom and fieldwork professional behaviors.

The high level of interrater reliability, internal consistency, and content validity established for this pilot version suggest that the scale items are easily measured and address the construct of EI. Further refinement of the actual question has the potential to produce an admission selection measure that can help occupational therapy programs more efficiently identify students with higher levels of EI.

Although we did not examine the use of the question and scale as an interview procedure, there may be potential for the instrument to be used in this way. There is some evidence that interview procedures are able to capture applicant EI more effectively than written essays due to the interviewer's ability to redirect applicants when they do not answer the question (Latif, 2004; Levashina et al., 2014; Pau et al., 2013). In our study we found that approximately one-third of applicants misinterpreted the question. Another third chose not to address the question and instead wrote about a subject of their own choosing. In an interview situation, such applicants could be redirected by the interviewer. Structured EI interviews—in which the interviewer asks structured questions about specific scenarios to yield EI information—have been found to be more time consuming than typical admission interviews because of the time needed to redirect applicants to address desired content (Levashina et al., 2014; Pau et al., 2013). In a high-stakes situation, such as a college interview, applicants may be more guarded and hesitant to talk about their experience of interpersonal conflict. The same may be true with the question when it is used in an essay format. In our study, two thirds of applicants wrote about situations they may have perceived as safe content for a college essay, such as experiencing an internal desire to change careers. It may be likely that students with lower levels of EI are less comfortable talking about their emotions and interpersonal conflict. Further testing of the conflict question used in a face-to-face interview may provide information about which format (essay or structured interview) yields greater information about an applicant's EI.

Limitations

One limitation of the study was the small sample size and predominance of white females as participants. Although the CUMC Occupational Therapy Program has a more diverse student population compared to the national average of occupational therapy schools (AOTA, 2014), our study sample nevertheless consisted largely of young adult white females. While our sample reflects the national average, having a more diverse sample would likely yield greater information about EI in student applicants. Although our expert panel rated the scale items as having high content validity, we only used three experts. Content validity would be stronger if repeated with 5 or more experts.

Future Research

While the initially established psychometric properties of the EI Admission Essay Scale were moderate to strong, we realize that the wording of our question must be made more specific and direct applicants to write about an interpersonal conflict. Once our question is rewritten for the subsequent scale version, it will be important to reassess psychometric properties. Future research is also needed to understand if the next scale version can discriminate between students with and without professional behavior problems in the academic and fieldwork settings.

Additional research could also be undertaken to understand if the question can be used in a structured admission interview format to yield information about applicant EI.

Summary

This study described the development of an admission essay scale designed to yield information about applicant EI and reported the scale's initial psychometric properties. Although initially established psychometric properties of the scale were moderate to strong, the wording of the essay question must be modified to help applicants focus their writing on interpersonal conflict. Despite the need for modification of question wording, findings of this study demonstrate that the EI Admission Essay Scale has the potential to be used as an admission selection criterion that can help occupational therapy programs better identify students with higher levels of EI.

References

American Occupational Therapy Association. (2002). *Fieldwork Performance Evaluation for the Occupational Therapy Student.* Bethesda, MD: AOTA Press.

American Occupational Therapy Association. (2014). *Academic Programs Annual Data Report: Academic Year 2013–2014.* Retrieved from http://www.aota.org//media/Corporate/Files/EducationCareers/Accredit/2013-2014-Annual-Data-Report.pdf

Arora, S., Ashrafian, H., Davis, R., Athanasiou, T., Darzi, A., & Sevdalis. (2010). Emotional intelligence in medicine: A systematic review through the context of the ACGME competencies. *Medical Education, 44,* 749–764. doi:10.1111/j.1365-2923.2010.03709.x

Bar-On, R. (1997). *The Emotional Quotient Inventory (EQ-i): A test of emotional intelligence.* Toronto: Multi-Health Systems.

Carr, S. E. (2009). Emotional intelligence in medical students: Does it correlate with selection measures? *Medical Education, 43*(11), 1069–1077. doi: 10.1111/j.1365-2923.2009.03496.x

Carrothers, R. M., Gregory, S. W., Jr., & Gallagher, T. J. (2000). Measuring emotional intelligence of medical school applicants. *Academic Medicine, 75*(5), 456–463. Retrieved from http://journals.lww.com/academicmedicine/Fulltext/2000/05000/Measuring_Emotional_Intelligence_of_Medical_School.16.aspx

Codier, E. E., Kofoed, N. A., & Peters, J. M. (2015). Graduate-entry non-nursing students: Is emotional intelligence the difference? *Nursing Education Perspectives, 36(*1), 46–47. doi:org/10.5480/12-874.1

DeVon, H. A., Block, M. E., Moyle-Wright, P., Ernst, D. M., Hayden, S. J., Lazzara, D. J., . . . & Kostas-Polston, E. (2007). A psychometric toolbox for testing validity and reliability. *Journal of Nursing Scholarship, 39*(2), 155–164. Retrieved from http://onlinelibrary.wiley.com/doi/10.1111/ j.1547-5069.2007.00161.x/pdf

Elam, C. L. (2000). Use of "emotional intelligence" as one measure of medical school applicants' noncognitive characteristics. *Academic Medicine, 75*(5), 445–446. Retrieved from http://journals. lww.com/academicmedicine/Fulltext/2000/05000/Use_of__Emotional_Intelligence__as_One_ Measure_of.11.aspx

Fiori, M., & Antonakis, J. (2011). The ability model of emotional intelligence: Searching for valid measures. *Personality and Individual Differences, 50*(3), 329–334. doi:10.1016/j.paid.2010.10.010

Hannah, A., Lim, B. T., & Ayers, K. M. (2009). Emotional intelligence and clinical interview performance of dental students. *Journal of Dental Education, 73*(9), 1107–1117. Retrieved from http:// www.jdentaled.org/content/73/9/1107.full.pdf+html

Jewell, R. T., McPherson, M. A., & Tieslau, M. A. (2013). Whose fault is it? Assigning blame for grade inflation in higher education. *Applied Economics, 45*(9), 1185–1200. doi: 10.1080/00036846.2011.621884

Jones-Schenk, J., & Harper, M. G. (2014). Emotional intelligence: An admission criterion alternative to cumulative grade point averages for prelicensure students. *Nurse Education Today, 34*(3), 413–420. doi:10.1016/j.nedt.2013.03.018

Latif, D. A. (2004). Using the structured interview for a more reliable assessment of pharmacy student applicants. *American Journal of Pharmaceutical Education, 68*(1), 1–7. doi: 10.5688/aj680121

Lawshe, C. H. (1975). A quantitative approach to content validity. *Personnel Psychology, 28*(4), 563–575. doi: 10.1111/j.1744-6570.1975.tb01393.x

Levashina, J., Hartwell, C. J., Morgeson, F. P., & Campion, M. A. (2014). The structured employment interview: Narrative and quantitative review of the research literature. *Personnel Psychology, 67*(1), 241–293. doi: 10.1111/peps.12052

Lyon, S. R., Trotter, F., Holt, B., Powell, E., & Roe, A. (2013). Emotional intelligence and its role in recruitment of nursing students. *Nursing Standard, 27*(40), 41-46. doi.org/10.7748/ns2013.06.27.40.41.e7529

Mayer, J. D., & Salovey, P. (1993). The intelligence of emotional intelligence. *Intelligence, 17*, 432–42. doi:10.1016/0160-2896(93)90010-3

McQueen, A. C. (2004). Emotional intelligence in nursing work. *Journal of Advanced Nursing, 47*(1), 101–108. doi: 10.1111/j.1365-2648.2004.03069.x

Pau, A., Jeevaratnam, K., Chen, Y. S., Fall, A. A., Khoo, C., & Nadarajah, V. D. (2013). The Multiple Mini-Interview (MMI) for student selection in health professions training–A systematic review. *Medical Teacher, 35*(12), 1027-1041. doi: 10.3109/0142159X.2013.829912

Portney, L. G., & Watkins, M. P. (2013). *Foundations of clinical research: Applications to practice* (3rd ed.). Upper Saddle River, NJ: Pearson, Prentice Hall.

Rankin, B. (2013). Emotional intelligence: Enhancing values-based practice and compassionate care in nursing. *Journal of Advanced Nursing, 69*(12), 2717-2725. doi: 10.1111/jan.12161

Romanelli, F., Cain, J., & Smith, K. M. (2006). Emotional intelligence as a predictor of academic and/or professional success. *American Journal of Pharmaceutical Education, 70*(3). doi: 10.5688/aj700369

Salovey, P., & Mayer, J. D. (1990). Emotional intelligence. *Imagination, Cognition, and Personality, 9*, 185–211. doi: 10.2190/DUGG-P24E-52WK-6CDG

Schutte, N. S., Malouff, J. M., & Bhullar, N. (2009). The Assessing Emotions Scale. In C. Stough, D. Saklofske, & J. Parker (Eds.), *The Assessment of Emotional Intelligence* (pp. 119–135). New York, NY: Springer.

Schutte, N. S., Malouff, J. M., Hall, L. E., Haggerty, D., J., Cooper, J. T., Golden, C. J., & Dornheim, L. (1998). Development and validation of a measure of emotional intelligence. *Personality and Individual Differences, 25*, 167–177. doi:10.1016/S0191-8869(98)00001-4

Victoroff, K. Z., & Boyatzis, R. E. (2013). What is the relationship between emotional intelligence and

dental student clinical performance? *Journal of Dental Education*, 77(4), 416-426. Retrieved from

http://www.jdentaled.org/content/77/4/416.full

REVIEWER COMMENTS WITH AUTHOR RESPONSES

Reviewer 1

Reviewer comment:

This paper provides a valuable addition to the literature and a thorough approach to establishing the validity of an instrument of measure. I am wondering about the statistical power of the findings, given the small N of 40. Usually a larger sample size is required to truly determine validity of an instrument. Please address this issue in your revision. Thank you.

Author response:

Thank you for bringing to our attention that we had not adequately addressed the issue relating to small sample size. We have revised our Limitations section as follows:

"One limitation of the study was the small sample size and predominance of white females as participants. Although the CUMC Occupational Therapy Program has a more diverse student population compared to the national average of occupational therapy schools (AOTA, 2014), our study sample nevertheless consisted largely of young adult white females. While our sample reflects the national average, having a more diverse and larger sample would likely yield greater information about EI in student applicants. A larger sample size would also enhance statistical power and rigor of results. Although our expert panel rated the scale items as having high content validity, we only used three experts. Content validity would be stronger if repeated with 5 or more experts."

Reviewer 2

Reviewer comment:

Overall this manuscript is well written and discusses an interesting topic, which is applied in a novel way to occupational therapy admission procedures. I appreciate the author's attempt to provide guidance for additional measures to be used for determination of admission into occupational therapy programs and the use of a non-academic-based criterion. Primary work on the establishment of an EI measure that is efficient, valid and reliable is useful and authors examined the psychometric properties in effective ways.

Some of the issues with this manuscript are that the concept of EI as an admission criterion needs to be further developed and supported. Although authors acknowledge EI is a skill, authors propose that it is essential applicants have high levels of EI before entering an occupational therapy program. The call for EI as an essential skill prior to beginning an occupational therapy course of study is not well supported by the literature review or author's findings.

Author response:

Thank you for helping us clarify that we have not suggested that student applicants must have high levels of EI before entering occupational therapy school. We are suggesting instead that an EI measure be used along with traditional cognitive and noncognitive measures to identify applicants with *higher* levels of EI—just as admission committees seek applicants with higher grades, more health- and occupational therapy-related experience, and greater diversity of life experience. We have added the following text to the paper in the Introduction section to address the reviewer's concerns:

"Occupational therapy is now ranked as the number ninth health care job by *US News and World Report* (2015) and applications to occupational therapy schools have more than doubled in the last decade (AOTA, 2014). Applicants who may not have the propensity for a health career but who are attracted to the job security and higher salaries that health careers provide have increasingly applied to health care schools in the last decade (Buerhaus, Auerbach, & Staiger, 2009). It has been the authors' experience that some students have professional behavioral problems related to emotional intelligence throughout the academic and fieldwork curricula. In the Occupational Therapy Program at Columbia University Medical Center (CUMC) we receive a high amount of applications and are only able to admit 10% of our applicant pool. Our desire to identify students with higher levels of emotional intelligence—and flag students who may not be adequately suited for an occupational therapy career—underpins our effort to develop an EI admission assessment that can be used adjunctly with traditional cognitive and noncognitive measures. Occupational therapy programs that identify students with limited emotional intelligence may prefer to help students develop EI in the occupational therapy curriculum."

Reviewer comment:

Introduction:

Authors did not adequately connect the main topic area (emotional intelligence) to the admission process. Additionally, EI is a skill and many health profession curricula include EI skills training. It was not made clear why this should be measured prior to admission and used as a selection criterion for entrance if it is something that can be taught and developed.

Authors state that the need for EI is elevated by the number of applicants, but it is not clear why the number of applicants increases the need for EI measures. Also authors make a statement about generational differences and values, but this also isn't clearly linked to the need for using EI measures in the admission process.

Author response:

As mentioned above, we have more fully addressed these points in the introduction with the following text:

"Occupational therapy program admission selection criteria have traditionally relied upon the cognitive measures of cumulative grade point average (GPA), prerequisite GPA, science GPA, and preadmission standardized tests such as the Graduate Record Exam (GRE) (Romanelli, Cain, & Smith, 2006). Traditionally used noncognitive measures have included interviews, personal statements and essays, volunteerism, and prior service and healthcare experience (Jones-Schenk & Harper, 2014). While the above cognitive and noncognitive measures have been shown to provide accurate predictive information about an applicant's academic performance in graduate school (Carr, 2009), they do not provide information about an applicant's potential clinical performance and professional behaviors in the academic program and fieldwork experiences. Given the large number of occupational therapy clinical competencies that relate to EI, it seems prudent to have an admission criterion that measures an applicant's EI and can identify students who have both the academic skill and EI needed to succeed in an occupational therapy program and career. The need for an EI measure in the admission selection process has been elevated by the growing number of occupational therapy school applications in the last decades (American Occupational Therapy Association [AOTA], 2014), the inflation of academic grades at the college and university level lessening the rigor of GPA as a reliable assessment measure (Jewell, McPherson, & Tieslau, 2013), and the generational difference in students applying to health care programs who may have values and professional behaviors that are incongruent with health care professions and who may be qualitatively different from applicants of past decades (Romanelli et al., 2006). Occupational therapy is now ranked as the number ninth health care job by US News and World Reports (2015), and applications to occupational therapy schools have more than doubled in the last decade (AOTA, 2014). Applicants who may not have the propensity for a health career but who are attracted to the job security and higher salaries that health careers provide, have increasingly applied to health care schools in the last decade (Buerhaus, Auerbach, & Staiger, 2009). It has been the authors' experience that some students have professional behavioral problems related to emotional intelligence throughout the academic and fieldwork curricula. In the Occupational Therapy Program at Columbia University Medical Center (CUMC) we receive a high amount of applications and are only able to admit 10% of our applicant pool. Our desire to identify students with higher levels of emotional intelligence—and flag students who may not be adequately suited for an occupational therapy career—underpins our effort to develop an EI admission assessment that can be used adjunctly with traditional cognitive and noncognitive measures. Occupational therapy programs that identify students with limited emotional intelligence may prefer to help students develop EI in the occupational therapy curriculum."

We have also added the following text in the introduction regarding the debate about whether EI is a fairly static personality trait or a skill that can be learned:

"Research examining EI is relatively new and debate exists regarding whether EI is a personality trait that can be shaped within a set of parameters rooted in genetics and environment, or whether EI is a skill that can be taught and learned without a ceiling for potential (Petrides & Furnham, 2001)."

Reviewer comment:

It appears some of the citations used in the third paragraph are from secondary sources.

Author response:

We reviewed all citations and references and all are primary sources.

Reviewer comment:

Methods:

Authors should consistently use acronyms (on p. 5 authors use "Emotional Intelligence" vs. EI that is used throughout paper).

Author response:

Thank you for helping us to catch this error. We have corrected all acronyms in the paper.

Reviewer comment:

On page 7, authors indicate that more interpersonal skills are rated because these skills underlie the majority of clinical professional behaviors. This statement should be supported with a research citation, or this concept should be explored earlier in the paper.

Author response:

Thank you for helping us to better support our arguments with published data. We have now added the following citations:

McQueen, 2004; Victoroff & Boyatzis, 2013.

Reviewer comment:

Under Phase 5: Identifying how students with demonstrated problematic professional behaviors were identified would be helpful. Also, the author indicated that withdrawing or failing FW resulted in being identified as a professional behavior problem, but withdrawals and failures are not always related to professional behaviors. Did authors review the reasons for withdrawal and failure to ensure they were professional behavior problems?

Author response:

In the original text we stated that we identified students with professional behavior problems in the academic and fieldwork settings by determining whether they had received professional development forms and counseling from advisors. Students who exhibited professional behavioral problems during fieldwork had received behavioral contracts (due to professional behavioral problems) or had failed fieldwork. All of this information was confirmed with faculty, fieldwork coordinators, and fieldwork supervisors.

"Students who were identified as having problematic professional behaviors in the academic setting had received professional development forms and counseling from advisors. Students identified as exhibiting problematic professional behaviors in the fieldwork setting (Level I or II) had received behavioral contracts or had been withdrawn from or failed fieldwork."

In the above reviewer comment, the reviewer requests information that was provided in the original text. Sometimes reviewers overlook information. Reviewing a manuscript of 25+ pages can be overwhelming, particularly when a manuscript includes a great deal of methodological steps and analysis. Rather than become defensive, we stated that this information was provided and offer the original text.

Reviewer comment:

A table demonstrating distribution of scores on the EI scale would be helpful to understand the scoring. From the description under Phase 5 it looks like there were many low scores or scores of zero. This information would be helpful earlier in relationship to the other statistical analysis.

Author response:

Thank you for this suggestion. We have added a table of raw scores to better help readers understand the data.

Reviewer comment:

Limitations:
Convergent validity: Second-year students completed the 2 measures at 2 different time points in the program. As noted earlier, EI can develop over time, and therefore second-year student ratings may have been influenced by passage of time and exposure to clinical settings/educational materials/life experiences. This might be listed as a limitation.

Author response:

Both second- and first-year students completed the two measures. Second-year students completed the Assessing Emotions Scale at the beginning of their second year (third semester of curriculum), while first-year students completed the Assessing Emotions Scale at the beginning of their first semester. We used a Mann Whitney to determine that there was no statistically significant difference between their Assessing Emotions Scale, despite time of completion. The following is an excerpt from the original paper:

"Data Collection: Both first and second year participating students completed the Assessing Emotions Scale during the same 1-month period; however, first year students completed the scale in the first semester of their academic program, while second year students completed the scale in the third semester of their academic program. To determine that length in the academic program did not influence student EI scores, we analyzed whether a statistically significant difference existed between first and second year student scores on both the EI Admission Essay Scale and the Assessing Emotions Scale."

"Results: The data from 27 first year and 13 second year students (N = 40; male = 7, female = 33; White = 31, Asian = 5, African American = 2, Native American = 1, Hispanic = 1) were used to establish convergent validity between the EI Admission Essay Scale and the Assessing Emotions Scale. Convergent validity between these two scales was found to be moderate at $r = .46$, $p < .02$. Because first and second year students completed the Assessing Emotions Scale at different times in their curricula, we used a Mann Whitney U test to examine whether first and second year students differed in their EI levels (Portney & Watkins, 2013). A difference found may have been attributed to year in program; however, no statistically significant difference was found between first and second year students on both their EI Admission Essay Scale scores and the Assessing Emotions Scale scores."

The above reviewer comment was another instance of a reviewer requesting information that was provided in the original text. Again, we simply stated that this information was provided and offered sections from the original paper.

Reviewer comment:

There appears to be a lack of variance in the EI Admission Essay scores, which can impact statistical analysis. Because no descriptive statistics are provided for the distribution of scores, it is difficult for the reader to determine if this is true. But, with 1/3 of respondents receiving "0" the analysis may have been impacted. This might be listed as a limitation.

Author Response:

Thank you for addressing this point. We have inserted a table of raw scores so that readers can better understand the data.

Reviewer comment:

Summary:

The author's last statement about using the scale in admission selection to help better identify students with higher levels of EI is not supported by the research outcomes and should be restated. Use of the essay did not yield differences between those with higher and lower EI and performance. Therefore, using EI scores during admissions to determine those with higher EI will not predict performance, and including it in the admission process is not supported.

Author Response:

Thank you for helping us to better report our data. We disagree with the reviewer's statement that the scale, in its present form, cannot yield information about an applicant's EI. The current version of the EI Admission Essay Scale is moderately correlated with the Assessing Emotions Scale indicating that it has potential to identify students with higher levels of EI. What it cannot do in its present form is discriminate between students with and without professional behavioral problems in the academic and fieldwork settings. We have revised the text in question to read as follows:

In this reviewer comment, the reviewer asserts that the assessment cannot yield differences between students with higher and lower emotional intelligence scores. This is an instance where we simply stated that we disagreed with the reviewer and her suggestion that the scale cannot discriminate between students with higher and lower EI. We explained that the scale is in fact moderately correlated with the Assessing Emotions Scale (and can differentiate between students with higher and lower EI levels), but at this point cannot discriminate between students with and without professional behavioral problems in the academic and fieldwork settings. We modified the summary paragraph to clarify this confusion and provided the text changes.

"This study described the development of an admission essay scale designed to yield information about applicant EI and reported the scale's initial psychometric properties. Although initially established psychometric properties of the scale were moderate to strong, the wording of the essay question must be modified to help applicants focus their writing on interpersonal conflict. Despite the need for modification of question wording, findings of this study demonstrate that the EI Admission Essay Scale, once revised, has potential to be used as an admission selection criterion that can help occupational therapy programs better identify students with higher levels of EI."

Reviewer comment:

Conceptually, using an EI scale may contribute to the overall picture of an applicant, but using EI in the admissions process as if it is a static personality trait may create barriers for applicants with fewer life experiences. EI can be taught, therefore the scale might aid in identifying students with low EI who will potentially have performance issues, and supplemental education can be provided to assist them in developing the needed EI skills. Nursing literature has some examples of EI curriculum.

The argument that these skills must be present upon admission is not clear given the literature review and evidence presented in this manuscript.

Author response:

We hope that we have addressed this point in the previous section—that we are not suggesting that applicants have high levels of EI before admissions. Rather we suggest that an EI Admission Essay Scale can be used as one measure to identify stronger applicants.

REVISED DRAFT

Running head: EMOTIONAL INTELLIGENCE ADMISSION ESSAY SCALE

Development and Psychometric Properties of the

Emotional Intelligence Admission Essay Scale

Sharon A. Gutman, PhD, OTR, FAOTA

Janet P. Falk-Kessler, EdD, OTR, FAOTA

Abstract

Objective: The purpose was to describe the development and psychometric properties of the Emotional Intelligence Admission Essay scale.

Methods: The authors developed an admission essay question and rating scale designed to provide information about applicants' emotional intelligence (EI). Content validity, convergent validity, interrater reliability, and internal consistency were established. The scale was also examined to determine if it could discriminate between students with and without professional behavior problems in the academic and fieldwork settings.

Results: Content validity was found to be high by a panel of three experts in EI (content validity index = 1.0). Convergent validity with the Assessing Emotions Scale was moderate ($r = .46, p < .02$). Interrater reliability between two trained faculty raters was high ($ICC = .91, p < .000$). Internal consistency of the scale was high with a Cronbach's alpha of .95. This version of the scale was not able to discriminate between students with and without professional behavior problems.

Conclusion: The moderate to strong psychometric properties suggest that the EI Admission Essay Scale has the ability to provide information about applicants' EI. The wording of the essay question must be modified to better instruct applicants to address interpersonal conflict.

Keywords: occupational therapy, admission selection, instrument development

Emotional intelligence (EI) is a form of social intelligence that involves the ability to recognize and appraise emotions in oneself and others, regulate and manage emotions in oneself and others, and use emotion based information to guide behavior and problem solving (Arora et al., 2010). The term was first developed by Salovey and Mayer (1990) who argued that EI was a distinct set of skills that were separate from personality traits and previously identified types of intelligence. Later researchers extended the definition of EI by dissecting the construct into inter- and intrapersonal intelligences wherein interpersonal intelligence involves the ability to accurately read and assess other's verbal and nonverbal expressions; easily build rapport with others using an open, compassionate countenance that demonstrates interest in others; and successfully diffuse and negotiate interpersonal conflict (Carrothers, Gregory, & Gallagher, 2000; McQueen, 2004). Intrapersonal intelligence involves the ability to recognize emotion in oneself and understand its origin, be aware of how one's emotions impact one's behaviors and influence others, and monitor and regulate one's emotions to enhance emotional stability and wellness (Elam, 2000; McQueen, 2004). Research examining EI is relatively new and debate exists regarding whether EI is a personality trait that can be shaped within a set of parameters rooted in genetics and environment, or whether EI is a skill that can be taught and learned without a ceiling for potential (Petrides & Furnham, 2001).

This sentence was added to the Introduction to address the reviewer concern that we had not clarified whether emotional intelligence is a skill that can be learned or an innate personality trait.

Emotional intelligence is a critical skill for occupational therapists and clinical competencies relating to EI involve the ability to collaboratively work with a team of health care professionals; identify and manage patient emotions to adeptly address patient concerns and needs; identify and manage team member emotions to promote patient advocacy and diffuse possible professional domain conflicts; communicate with patients, family members, caregivers, health care providers, and insurers to ensure optimal patient care; educate caregivers who may feel overwhelmed and ill-prepared to assume caregiving responsibilities; and work cooperatively and compassionately with people from varied and diverse cultural groups (McQueen, 2004; Victoroff & Boyatzis, 2013). Given the great extent of clinical competencies that directly relate to emotional intelligence, it is surprising that this construct has not been formally examined in occupational therapy admission selection criteria.

Occupational therapy program admission selection criteria have traditionally relied upon the cognitive measures of cumulative grade point average (GPA), prerequisite GPA, science GPA, and preadmission standardized tests such as the Graduate Record Exam (GRE) (Romanelli, Cain, & Smith, 2006). Traditionally used noncognitive measures have included interviews, personal statements and essays, volunteerism, and prior service and healthcare experience (Jones-Schenk & Harper, 2014). While the above cognitive and noncognitive measures have been shown to provide accurate predictive information about an applicant's academic performance in graduate school (Carr, 2009), they do not provide information about an applicant's potential clinical performance and professional behaviors in the academic program and fieldwork experiences. Given the large number of occupational therapy clinical competencies that relate to EI, it seems prudent to have an admission criterion that measures an applicant's EI and can identify students who have both the academic skill and EI needed to succeed in an occupational therapy program and career. The need for an EI measure in the admission selection process has been elevated by the growing number of occupational therapy school applications in the last decades (American Occupational Therapy Association [AOTA], 2014), the inflation of academic grades at the college and university level lessening the rigor of GPA as a reliable assessment measure (Jewell, McPherson, & Tieslau, 2013), and the generational difference in students applying to health care programs who may have values and professional behaviors that are incongruent with health care professions and who may be qualitatively different from applicants of past decades (Romanelli et al., 2006). Occupational therapy is now ranked as the number ninth health care job by US News and World Reports (2015) and applications to occupational therapy schools have more than doubled in the last decade (AOTA, 2014). Applicants who may not have the propensity for a health career but who are attracted to the job security and higher salaries that health careers provide, have increasingly applied to health care schools in the last decade (Buerhaus, Auerbach, & Staiger, 2009). It has been the authors' experience that some students have professional behavioral problems related to emotional intelligence throughout the academic and fieldwork curricula. In the Occupational Therapy Program at Columbia University Medical Center (CUMC) we receive a high amount of applications and are only able to admit 10% of our applicant pool. Our desire to identify students with higher levels of emotional intelligence–and flag students who may not be adequately suited for an occupational therapy career–underpins our effort to develop an EI admission assessment that can be used adjunctly with traditional cognitive and noncognitive measures. Occupational therapy programs that identify students with limited emotional intelligence may prefer to help students develop EI in the occupational therapy curriculum.

These sentences were added or refined from the original text in response to the reviewer's concern that we had not adequately argued that emotional intelligence is an essential admission criterion. We specifically inserted the final sentence in this paragraph to address the reviewer's concern that some students may be able to enhance their emotional intelligence through coursework in the curriculum.

Other health care professions have begun to recognize the value of using EI measures in the admission selection process. Much of the literature addressing the EI of health care student applicants has been generated by the professions of medicine, nursing, dentistry, and pharmacy (Arora, et al., 2010; Lyon, Trotter, Holt, Powell, & Roe 2013; Victoroff & Boyatzis, 2013; Romanelli et al., 2006). These studies have found that students with high levels of EI as measured on standardized assessments demonstrate higher levels of clinical performance (Codier, Kofoed, & Peters, 2015; Hannah, Lim, & Ayers, 2009; Rankin, 2013), are more highly rated by clinical supervisors and patients (Arora et al., 2010; Hannah et al., 2009; Rankin, 2013; Victoroff & Boyatzis, 2013), are more likely to complete their professional health care education programs (Jones-Schenk & Harper, 2014; Rankin, 2013), and are better able to work collaboratively on treatment teams as assessed by supervisors (Arora et al., 2010; Victoroff & Boyatzis, 2013). Most of the EI measures used in these studies were administered to students already matriculated in health care programs and all authors supported the need for the incorporation of EI measures administered during the admission process.

Although the need for and value of EI measures used during the admission selection process of health care programs is clear, the most practical and reliable type of EI measure is of debate. The most commonly available form of EI measure is a paper and pencil or computer generated test (Arora et al., 2010). Such assessments either pose scenarios and ask respondents to identify the most emotionally intelligent answer through a multiple choice format or are self-report measures that ask respondents to identify to what extent they identify with a specific skill (e.g., "I am able to read other's facial expressions to determine their mood.") (Fiori & Antonakis, 2011). Another form of EI assessment gaining interest among health care programs is the structured interview, in which a specific set of questions is asked of all applicants (Latif, 2004; Levashina, Hartwell, Morgeson, & Campion, 2014; Pau et al., 2013). In the structured interview, applicants may be consecutively interviewed by several interviewers who are all trained in interview administration and have established interrater reliability in the use of a standardized EI rating scale. While the use of face-to-face structured interviews and standardized paper and pencil or computer generated tests are often reliable and valid, they can be costly and labor intensive. Most EI measures with established reliability and validity are expensive and an administration fee is charged per student. Structured interviewing is time and labor intensive and requires training interviewers in both administration and assessment.

> A reviewer found that we had spelled out "emotional intelligence" and helped us to recheck all EI acronyms in the paper.

In response to the need to incorporate a practical and reliable EI measure into the admission selection process, the faculty in the Occupational Therapy Program at CUMC have developed an essay question and rating scale, the EI Admission Essay Scale, which may have the ability to provide information about an applicant's EI. The essay question asks applicants to describe a conflict situation in a work, school, or personal event; how the applicant knowingly or unknowingly contributed to the conflict; and how he or she attempted to resolve the conflict based on the ability to use emotion based information to guide problem solving. The instrument used to assess the applicant's essay is a 5-item, 4-point Likert scale with a range from 0 (no evidence) to 3 (strong evidence). The purpose of the present study was to develop the pilot version of the EI Admission Essay Scale, and establish content and convergent validity, interrater reliability, and internal consistency. Additionally, we hoped to determine whether the scale is able to discriminate between students who have professional behavior problems in the academic and fieldwork setting and students who do not.

The research questions were:

1. Can an admission essay question and rating scale be developed to provide information about an applicant's EI?

2. Using a panel of three experts in emotional intelligence research, what is the content validity of the EI Admission Essay Scale?

3. Does the EI Admission Essay Scale have convergent validity with the Assessing Emotions Scale (Schutte et al., 1998; Schutte, Malouff, & Bhullar, 2009)?

4. Using trained occupational therapy faculty raters, can interrater reliability be established for the EI Admission Essay Scale?

5. What is the internal consistency of the EI Admission Essay Scale using data from first year students in the CUMC Occupational Therapy Entry-Level Program?

6. Can the EI Admission Essay Scale discriminate between students who have professional behavior problems in the academic and/or fieldwork setting and students who do not?

Method

Research Design

This study described the development of a pilot assessment intended to measure EI in occupational therapy program applicants. Psychometric properties of the pilot instrument that were established included content and convergent validity, interrater reliability, and internal consistency as described below. We additionally examined whether the EI Admission Essay Scale could discriminate between students with and without professional behavior problems. The CUMC IRB approved this study and all participants provided consent.

Phase 1: Content Validity

Participants. To establish content validity of the EI Admission Essay Scale we assembled a panel of three professionals having expertise in EI research and literature. One expert was a physician educator who developed and implemented admission interview procedures for medical school applicants to ascertain information about EI. A second expert was a director of student wellness at a large, urban, northeastern university and specialized in emotional intelligence. A third expert was a professor in the Center for Educational Research and Evaluation at CUMC and taught coursework in EI.

Procedures. To develop the essay question and rating scale, the authors completed a literature review of EI research and divided the construct into its component parts of intra- and interpersonal intelligence. Since successful conflict negotiation is a key determinant of higher levels of EI (McQueen, 2004; & Boyatzis, 2013), we developed a question in which applicants were asked to describe a conflict situation that occurred in a work, school, or personal situation. To gain insight into the applicant's awareness of ways in which his or her behavior and emotions impacted others (intrapersonal intelligence), applicants were asked to describe how they may have knowingly or unknowingly contributed to the conflict. To gain information about the applicant's ability to consider others' emotions and work collaboratively (interpersonal intelligence), we then asked applicants to describe their attempts at conflict resolution. Applicants were asked to address this question in 750 words. The question read as follows: "Describe a conflict that existed in a class, job, or life event in which you were a participant. How did you contribute wittingly or unwittingly to this conflict? How was the conflict handled by all involved parties?"

To develop a rating scale that could evaluate the EI content of the essay, we returned to our list of component parts of EI and formulated five scale items that addressed both intra- and interpersonal intelligence as described below. The scale items more heavily focus on interpersonal skills since such skills underlie a majority of clinical professional behaviors (McQueen, 2004; Victoroff & Boyatzis, 2013).

> We added these citations to support the assertion that interpersonal skills underlie a majority of clinical professional behaviors, as requested by one reviewer.

1. The applicant was able to place self in others' shoes to understand others' experiences, emotions, and perspectives in a conflict situation. (Interpersonal intelligence)

2. The applicant was able to understand how one's own actions contributed to a conflict. (Intrapersonal intelligence)

3. The applicant attempted to understand the conflict situation without blaming others for the conflict. (Interpersonal intelligence)

4. The applicant attempted to create a resolution that benefited all parties of a conflict to the greatest extent possible. (Interpersonal intelligence)

5. The applicant was able to cooperate equally with others in a conflict situation to problem solve and form a resolution to the conflict (i.e., did not monopolize problem solving or present oneself as hero). (Interpersonal intelligence)

Data collection. Expert raters were then provided with the essay question, list of scale items, and a rating scale form and were asked to complete and return the rating form via email. Experts did not consult with one another or have access to each other's scores.

Data analysis. We then completed a content validity ratio (CVR) (Lawshe, 1975) by asking the three experts to determine whether each scale item was congruent with the construct of EI. Experts rated each scale item using a three-point scale where 0 = not essential, 1 = useful, and 2 = essential. The CVR for each item was calculated using the formula below where ne is the number of experts who rated the item as essential and N is the total number of experts.

$$CVR = \frac{ne - N/2}{N/2}$$

A content validity index (CVI), the score for the entire instrument, was then calculated by determining the mean for all retained items (Lawshe suggests that items receiving a 0 be discarded). Using a content validity index, items require a .83 level of endorsement to establish content validity (DeVon et al., 2007); however, if 4 or fewer raters are used, the CVR for each item must be 1 to demonstrate content validity.

After content validity was established for the five scale items, we developed a 4-point rating scale for all items where 0 = no evidence, 1 = minimal evidence, 2 = moderate evidence, and 3 = strong evidence. Possible total scores range from 0 to 15 with higher scores indicating higher EI.

Results. All three experts rated each of the five essay scale items as essential (2.0) which resulted in a CVR of 1.0 for each item and a CVI of 1.0 for the entire scale. As a result, this pilot version of the scale was determined to have high content validity with the construct of EI.

Phase 2: Convergent Validity

Participants. To enroll in this study participants had to be matriculated first or second year students in the CUMC Occupational Therapy Entry-Level Program who completed the EI Admission Essay Scale as part of their application process. Participation was voluntary and students could choose not to participate. Students were recruited through an email invitation with an embedded link to an online version of the Assessing Emotions Scale (Schutte et al., 1998, 2009). We retrospectively collected admission essay questions of applicants enrolled as current first and second year students.

Procedures. To establish convergent validity we correlated EI Admission Essay Scale scores of 40 first and second year students with their scores on the Assessing Emotions Scale (Schutte et al., 1998, 2009). The Assessing Emotions Scale is a self-report measure of EI based on Salovey and Mayer's (1990) original model of EI (Mayer & Salovey, 1993). The scale has 33 items, uses a 5-point scale (1 = strongly disagree, 2 = somewhat disagree, 3 = neither agree nor disagree, 4 = somewhat agree, 5 = strongly agree), and requires approximately 5 minutes to complete. Total scores range from 33 to 165 with higher scores indicating higher levels of EI. Internal consistency of the scale was reported to be high with a Cronbach's alpha of .90 (Schutte et al., 1998, 2009). Schutte also reported that test-retest reliability was moderately high ($r = .78$, $p < .05$). Convergent validity with the Emotional Quotient Inventory (Bar-On, 1997) was found to be moderate ($r = .43$, $p < .05$) (Schutte et al., 1998, 2009).

Data collection. Both first and second year participating students completed the Assessing Emotions Scale during the same 1-month period; however, first year students completed the scale in the first semester of their academic program, while second year students completed the scale in the third semester of their academic program. To determine that length in the academic program did not influence student EI scores, we analyzed whether a statistically significant difference existed between first and second year student scores on both the EI Admission Essay Scale and the Assessing Emotions Scale.

The essay questions, which had been completed as part of the application process, were retrieved from student files by an admissions coordinator who coded and masked them. Students completed the Assessing Emotions Scale anonymously using their university ID numbers as codes. The master list linking codes to student names was maintained electronically on a password protected and encrypted computer by the admissions coordinator.

Both authors rated all 40 student EI Admission Essay Scales, first separately and then together to establish consensus when disagreement occurred. All essays were masked and authors were blinded to each other's initial scores. Interrater reliability between both authors was found to be high for separate, blinded ratings ($ICC = .94$, $p < .01$).

Data analysis. Data were entered into SPSS version 21 and level of significance was set at .05. To determine if EI Admission Essay Scale scores correlated with scores of the Assessing Emotions Scale, a Spearman rho correlation coefficient was used (Portney & Watkins, 2013).

Results. The data from 27 first year and 13 second year students (N = 40; male = 7, female = 33; White = 31, Asian = 5, African American = 2, Native American = 1, Hispanic = 1) were used to establish convergent validity between the EI Admission Essay Scale and the Assessing Emotions Scale. Convergent validity between these two scales was found to be moderate at $r = .46$, $p < .02$. Because first and second year students completed the Assessing Emotions Scale at different times in their curricula, we used a Mann Whitney U test to examine whether first and second year students differed in their EI levels (Portney & Watkins, 2013). A difference found may have been attributed to year in program; however, no statistically significant difference was found between first and second year students on both their EI Admission Essay Scale scores and the Assessing Emotions Scale scores.

Phase 3: Interrater Reliability

Participants. To establish interrater reliability of the EI Admission Essay Scale, two faculty members of the CUMC Occupational Therapy Program volunteered to serve as raters. These faculty members responded to an email invitation sent by the first author to all 10 full-time faculty members of the CUMC Occupational Therapy Program.

Procedures. The two faculty members received one hour of training in EI Admission Essay Scale rating procedures; training was provided by the first author. After training, raters were asked to separately rate three masked essays randomly selected from the total pool of 54 essays submitted by the first year class; essays were randomly selected by authors using a table of random numbers.

Data collection. The raters' scores for the three essays were completed separately and submitted by email one day after their training period. Raters were blinded to each other's scores.

Data analysis. Data were entered into SPSS version 21 and level of significance was set at .05. An intraclass correlation coefficient was used to determine interrater reliability between the two trained raters (Portney & Watkins, 2013).

Results. Interrater reliability was found to be high ($ICC = .91, p < .000$).

Phase 4: Internal Consistency

Participants. To determine the internal consistency of the EI Admission Essay Scale, we used the retrospectively collected admission essays of the 54 applicants admitted as current first year students (male = 10, female = 44; White = 44, Asian = 4, African American = 4, two or more races = 3).

Procedures. The essays of the 54 matriculated first year students were retrieved by the admissions coordinator who masked and coded them. Authors had already rated all essays during the procedures used to establish convergent validity. As stated above, essays were rated by both authors, first separately while blinded to each other's scores, and then together to address the existence of differences until consensus was reached. Achieving consensus was important to create one score for each essay item so that internal consistency could be determined. Interrater reliability between both authors for blinded rating was high ($ICC = .94, p < .01$). After the essays of all 54 first year students were rated by both authors and one score was established for each item (for all essays), the item scores for all essays were compared to determine internal consistency.

Data collection. Students completed the EI essays approximately 6 to 8 months earlier as part of their admissions application. This data set was retrospectively collected for this study by the admissions coordinator. Essays were masked and authors were blinded to each other's scores in the initial phase of rating.

Data analysis. Data were entered into SPSS version 21 and level of significance was set at .05. To determine if a correlation existed between scale items, a Cronbach's alpha correlation coefficient was used (Portney & Watkins, 2013).

Results. Internal consistency was found to be high with a Cronbach's alpha of .95.

Phase 5: Discrimination between Problematic and Nonproblematic Students

Participants. Data were the retrospectively collected admission essays of 54 admitted first year students.

Procedures. One objective of this study was to determine if the EI Admission Essay Scale could discriminate between students who demonstrated professional behavior problems in the academic and fieldwork environments and those who did not. We decided not to determine if EI Admission Essay Scale scores correlated with student scores on the American Occupational Therapy Association (AOTA) Fieldwork Evaluation (AOTA, 2002) because raters of the AOTA assessment had not attained interrater reliability with each other. Instead, we first identified those students who demonstrated problematic professional behaviors in the academic and fieldwork environments and then determined if a statistically significant difference existed between their EI Admission Essay Scale scores and the scores of students who did not demonstrate professional behavior problems. Students who were identified as having problematic professional behaviors in the academic setting had received professional development forms and counseling from advisors. Students identified as exhibiting problematic professional behaviors in the fieldwork setting (Level I or II) had received behavioral contracts or had been withdrawn from or failed fieldwork.

Data collection. Data used to determine whether EI Admission Essay Scale scores could discriminate between problematic and nonproblematic students were the student EI Admission Essay Scale scores, student records of professional development forms (indicating that the student was counseled by the academic advisor as a result of problematic professional behaviors), and documentation of fieldwork behavioral contracts or withdrawal/failure. Examining whether the EI Admission Essay Scale could discriminate between students with and without professional behavior problems required that we unmask and link essays with academic and fieldwork performance information. For this reason, we completed this step as a final study activity to avoid biasing the procedures used to establish convergent validity, interrater reliability, and internal consistency.

Data analysis. To determine if the EI Admission Essay Scale could discriminate between students who experienced professional behavior problems and those who did not, we used a Mann Whitney U test (Portney & Watkins, 2013).

Results. Five students demonstrated problematic professional behavior in the academic and fieldwork settings during the first year curriculum. A Mann Whitney U test showed no statistically significant difference between the EI Admission Essay Scale scores of these 5 students and the remaining 49 of the first year class. Despite a lack of statistical significance, however, it is interesting to note that these five students all obtained scores of 0 on their EI Admission Essay Scales, indicating the lowest possible score. Other students, however, also obtained 0 scores because they either failed to answer the question or showed no evidence of EI in their essays. When examining the 54 essays as a whole we found that only 18 (33.33%) answered the question and wrote about an experience of interpersonal conflict. Sixteen (29.62%) misinterpreted the question and wrote about an internal conflict that did not involve the ability to interpret and address others' emotions; 20 (37.03%) did not answer the question and wrote about their background, achievements, and career goals (see Table 9-1). Because of the large number of students who did not adequately answer the question and received low or 0 scores, it was difficult to statistically discriminate between students who possessed professional behavior problems and those who did not.

Discussion

This study aimed to determine if an admission essay scale could be developed that could capture information about an applicant's EI. The study also sought to establish the psychometric properties of content validity, convergent validity, interrater reliability, and internal consistency for this pilot version of the EI Admission Essay Scale. Because high content validity was established with a panel of experts and moderate convergent validity was found between the EI Admission Essay Scale and the Assessing Emotions Scale, we suggest that the EI Admission Essay Scale can yield information about an applicant's EI.

Although we hoped that the EI Admission Essay Scale could discriminate between students with and without professional behavior problems, we found that this version of the essay question was not able to do so, primarily because a large number of student applicants misinterpreted the question and wrote about an internal conflict rather than an interpersonal one. Although student essays addressing internal conflicts did provide some information about EI, essay content failed to address information about interpersonal intelligence. We realize that our question must be rewritten to provide clearer instructions about required essay content, particularly addressing interpersonal conflict. Once the question is rewritten we believe that the essay will have greater potential to yield information about EI and possibly predictive validity with classroom and fieldwork professional behaviors.

The high level of interrater reliability, internal consistency, and content validity established for this pilot version suggest that the scale items are easily measured and address the construct of EI.

Further refinement of the actual question has the potential to produce an admission selection measure that can help occupational therapy programs more efficiently identify students with higher levels of EI.

Although we did not examine the use of the question and scale as an interview procedure, there may be potential for the instrument to be used in this way. There is some evidence that interview procedures are able to capture applicant EI more effectively than written essays due to the interviewer's ability to redirect applicants when they do not answer the question (Latif, 2004; Levashina et al., 2014; Pau et al., 2013). In our study we found that approximately one-third of applicants misinterpreted the question. Another third chose not to address the question and instead wrote about a subject of their own choosing. In an interview situation, such applicants could be redirected by the interviewer. Structured EI interviews—in which the interviewer asks structured questions about specific scenarios to yield EI information—have been found to be more time consuming than typical admission interviews because of the time needed to redirect applicants to address desired content (Levashina et al., 2014; Pau et al., 2013). In a high-stakes situation, such as a college interview, applicants may be more guarded and hesitant to talk about their experience of interpersonal conflict. The same may be true with the question when it is used in an essay format. In our study, two thirds of applicants wrote about situations they may have perceived as safe content for a college essay, such as experiencing an internal desire to change careers. It may be likely that students with lower levels of EI are less comfortable talking about their emotions and interpersonal conflict. Further testing of the conflict question used in a face-to-face interview may provide information about which format (essay or structured interview) yields greater information about an applicant's EI.

> The Limitation section was revised to better address the study's small sample size.

Limitations

One limitation of the study was the small sample size and predominance of white females as participants. Although the CUMC Occupational Therapy Program has a more diverse student population compared to the national average of occupational therapy schools (AOTA, 2014), our study sample nevertheless consisted largely of young adult white females. While our sample reflects the national average, having a more diverse and larger sample would likely yield greater information about EI in student applicants. A larger sample size would also enhance statistical power and rigor of results. Although our expert panel rated the scale items as having high content validity, we only used three experts. Content validity would be stronger if repeated with 5 or more experts.

Future Research

While the initially established psychometric properties of the EI Admission Essay Scale were moderate to strong, we realize that the wording of our question must be made more specific and direct applicants to write about an interpersonal conflict. Once our question is rewritten for the subsequent scale version, it will be important to reassess psychometric properties. Future research is also needed to understand if the next scale version can discriminate between students with and without professional behavior problems in the academic and fieldwork settings. Additional research could also be undertaken to understand if the question can be used in a structured admission interview format to yield information about applicant EI.

Summary

This study described the development of an admission essay scale designed to yield information about applicant EI and reported the scale's initial psychometric properties. Although initially established psychometric properties of the scale were moderate to strong, the wording of the essay question must be modified to help applicants focus their writing on interpersonal conflict. Despite the need for modification of question wording, findings of this study demonstrate that the EI Admission Essay Scale, once revised, has potential to be used as an admission selection criterion that can help occupational therapy programs better identify students with higher levels of EI.

To address a reviewer concern, we modified the summary paragraph to emphasize that although the current version of the instrument can identify students with higher levels of EI, problems in the essay question wording must be revised before the scale can be used as an admission instrument.

References

American Occupational Therapy Association. (2002). *Fieldwork Performance Evaluation for the Occupational Therapy Student.* Bethesda, MD: AOTA Press.

American Occupational Therapy Association. (2014). *Academic Programs Annual Data Report: Academic Year 2013–2014.* Retrieved from http://www.aota.org//media/Corporate/Files/ EducationCareers/Accredit/2013-2014-Annual-Data-Report.pdf

Arora, S., Ashrafian, H., Davis, R., Athanasiou, T., Darzi, A., & Sevdalis. (2010). Emotional intelligence in medicine: A systematic review through the context of the ACGME competencies. *Medical Education, 44,* 749–764. doi:10.1111/j.1365-2923.2010.03709.x

Bar-On, R. (1997). *The Emotional Quotient Inventory (EQ-i):* A test of emotional intelligence. Toronto: Multi-Health Systems.

Buerhaus, P. I., Auerbach, D. I., & Staiger, D. O. (2009). The recent surge in nurse employment: Causes and implications. *Health Affairs, 28*(4), w657–w668. doi: 10.1377/hlthaff.28.4.w657

Carr, S. E. (2009). Emotional intelligence in medical students: Does it correlate with selection measures? *Medical Education, 43*(11), 1069–1077. doi: 10.1111/j.1365-2923.2009.03496.x

Carrothers, R. M., Gregory, S. W., Jr., & Gallagher, T. J. (2000). Measuring emotional intelligence of medical school applicants. *Academic Medicine, 75*(5), 456–463. Retrieved from http://journals. lww.com/academicmedicine/Fulltext/2000/05000/ Measuring_Emotional_Intelligence_of_ Medical_School.16.aspx

Codier, E. E., Kofoed, N. A., & Peters, J. M. (2015). Graduate-entry non-nursing students: Is emotional intelligence the difference? *Nursing Education Perspectives, 36*(1), 46–47. doi:org/10.5480/12-874.1

DeVon, H. A., Block, M. E., Moyle-Wright, P., Ernst, D. M., Hayden, S. J., Lazzara, D. J., . . . & Kostas-Polston, E. (2007). A psychometric toolbox for testing validity and reliability. *Journal of Nursing Scholarship, 39*(2), 155–164. Retrieved from http://onlinelibrary.wiley.com/doi/10.1111/ j.1547-5069.2007.00161.x/pdf

Elam, C. L. (2000). Use of "emotional intelligence" as one measure of medical school applicants' noncognitive characteristics. *Academic Medicine, 75*(5), 445–446. Retrieved from http://journals. lww.com/academicmedicine/Fulltext/2000/05000/Use_of__Emotional_ Intelligence__as_One_ Measure_of.11.aspx

Fiori, M., & Antonakis, J. (2011). The ability model of emotional intelligence: Searching for valid measures. *Personality and Individual Differences, 50*(3), 329–334. doi:10.1016/j.paid.2010.10.010

Hannah, A., Lim, B. T., & Ayers, K. M. (2009). Emotional intelligence and clinical interview performance of dental students. *Journal of Dental Education, 73*(9), 1107–1117. Retrieved from http:// www.jdentaled.org/content/73/9/1107.full.pdf+html

Jewell, R. T., McPherson, M. A., & Tieslau, M. A. (2013). Whose fault is it? Assigning blame for grade inflation in higher education. *Applied Economics, 45*(9), 1185–1200. doi: 10.1080/00036846.2011.621884

Jones-Schenk, J., & Harper, M. G. (2014). Emotional intelligence: An admission criterion alternative to cumulative grade point averages for prelicensure students. *Nurse Education Today, 34*(3), 413–420. doi:10.1016/j.nedt.2013.03.018

Latif, D. A. (2004). Using the structured interview for a more reliable assessment of pharmacy student applicants. *American Journal of Pharmaceutical Education, 68*(1), 1–7. doi: 10.5688/aj680121

Lawshe, C. H. (1975). A quantitative approach to content validity. *Personnel Psychology, 28*(4), 563–575. doi: 10.1111/j.1744-6570.1975.tb01393.x

Levashina, J., Hartwell, C. J., Morgeson, F. P., & Campion, M. A. (2014). The structured employment interview: Narrative and quantitative review of the research literature. *Personnel Psychology, 67*(1), 241–293. doi: 10.1111/peps.12052

Lyon, S. R., Trotter, F., Holt, B., Powell, E., & Roe, A. (2013). Emotional intelligence and its role in recruitment of nursing students. *Nursing Standard, 27*(40), 41–46. doi.org/10.7748/ ns2013.06.27.40.41.e7529

Mayer, J. D., & Salovey, P. (1993). The intelligence of emotional intelligence. *Intelligence, 17*, 432–42. doi:10.1016/0160-2896(93)90010-3

McQueen, A. C. (2004). Emotional intelligence in nursing work. *Journal of Advanced Nursing, 47*(1), 101–108. doi: 10.1111/j.1365-2648.2004.03069.x

Pau, A., Jeevaratnam, K., Chen, Y. S., Fall, A. A., Khoo, C., & Nadarajah, V. D. (2013). The Multiple Mini-Interview (MMI) for student selection in health professions training–A systematic review. *Medical Teacher, 35*(12), 1027–1041. doi: 10.3109/0142159X.2013.829912

Petrides, K. V., & Furnham, A. (2001). Trait emotional intelligence: Psychometric investigation with reference to established trait taxonomies. *European Journal of Personality, 15*(6), 425–448. doi: 10.1002/per.416

Portney, L. G., & Watkins, M. P. (2013). *Foundations of clinical research: Applications to practice* (3rd ed.). Upper Saddle River, NJ: Pearson, Prentice Hall.

Rankin, B. (2013). Emotional intelligence: Enhancing values-based practice and compassionate care in nursing. *Journal of Advanced Nursing, 69*(12), 2717–2725. doi: 10.1111/jan.12161

Romanelli, F., Cain, J., & Smith, K. M. (2006). Emotional intelligence as a predictor of academic and/or professional success. *American Journal of Pharmaceutical Education, 70*(3). doi: 10.5688/aj700369

Salovey, P., & Mayer, J. D. (1990). *Emotional intelligence. Imagination, Cognition, and Personality, 9,* 185–211. doi: 10.2190/DUGG-P24E-52WK-6CDG

Schutte, N. S., Malouff, J. M., & Bhullar, N. (2009). The Assessing Emotions Scale. In C. Stough, D. Saklofske, & J. Parker (Eds.), *The Assessment of Emotional Intelligence* (pp. 119–135). New York, NY: Springer.

Schutte, N. S., Malouff, J. M., Hall, L. E., Haggerty, D., J., Cooper, J. T., Golden, C. J., & Dornheim, L. (1998). Development and validation of a measure of emotional intelligence. *Personality and Individual Differences, 25,* 167–177. doi:10.1016/S0191-8869(98)00001-4

US News and World Report. (2015). Best health care jobs. Retrieved from http://money.usnews.com/careers/best-jobs/rankings/best-healthcare-jobs

Victoroff, K. Z., & Boyatzis, R. E. (2013). What is the relationship between emotional intelligence and dental student clinical performance? *Journal of Dental Education, 77*(4), 416–426. Retrieved from http://www.jdentaled.org/content/77/4/416.full

A table of raw scores was added at the request of one reviewer.

Table 1

Distribution of EI Admission Essay Scale Scores

Participant	EI Admission Essay Scale Score	Participant	EI Admission Essay Scale Score
1	14*	28	1**
2	13*	29	1**
3	13*	30	1**
4	12*	31	0**
5	11*	32	0**
6	11*	33	0**
7	10*	34	0**
8	10*	35	0***
9	9*	36	0***
10	7*	37	0***
11	6*	38	0***
12	6*	39	0***
13	3*	40	0***
14	3*	41	0***
15	2*	42	0***
16	2*	43	0***
17	2*	44	0***
18	2*	45	0***
19	2**	46	0***
20	2**	47	0***
21	2**	48	0***
22	1**	49	0***
23	1**	50	0***
24	1**	51	0***
25	1**	52	0***
26	1**	53	0***
27	1**	54	0***

Note: *Indicates scores of applicants (n = 18, 33.33%) who answered the question and wrote about an experience of interpersonal conflict. **Indicates scores of applicants (n = 16, 29.62%) who misinterpreted the question and wrote about an internal conflict that did not involve the ability to interpret and address others' emotions. ***Indicates scores of applicants (n = 20, 37.03%) who did not answer the question and wrote about their background, achievements, and career goals.

CHECKLIST FOR THE REVISION PROCESS

- ☐ Understand that revision is part of the journal submission process.

- ☐ Depersonalize reviewer feedback by separating emotional reactions from reviewer comments that can strengthen the manuscript. Set aside reviewer feedback for a few days until emotional reactions are no longer experienced.

- ☐ Begin to generate ideas for incorporating requested revisions into the next manuscript draft.

- ☐ If uncertainty exists regarding the meaning of reviewer feedback for a specific item, first consult with coauthors and colleagues. The editor should be contacted directly if a specific reviewer comment cannot be interpreted.

- ☐ Once all reviewer comments are understood, identify those revisions that will be addressed and generate ideas about how revisions will be made.

- ☐ Estimate the time needed for revisions, develop a timeline, and adhere to it so that the manuscript can be resubmitted by the appointed due date.

- ☐ Make sure to adhere to the journal's specified word and page counts during the revision process.

- ☐ When the revised manuscript is complete, generate the document listing responses to reviewer comments. List all reviewer comments followed by complete and clear author responses.

- ☐ In the document listing responses to reviewer comments, justify the decision to omit certain reviewer recommendations with a clear explanation that is free from emotional language.

- ☐ Use neutral, positive language in all correspondence and in the responses to reviewer comments.

- ☐ Thank the editor and reviewers for their help in all correspondence and in the document listing responses to reviewer comments.

- ☐ Thoroughly proof the revised manuscript to identify and correct grammatical and stylistic errors, inconsistencies between citations and references, and inconsistencies between text and tables.

- ☐ Once the manuscript is resubmitted, use the journal's online tracking system to determine the status of a manuscript review. Do not contact the editor until 1 month has expired beyond the allotted review time.

REFERENCE

Gutman, S. A., & Falk-Kessler, J. P. (2016). Development and psychometric properties of the Emotional Intelligence Admission Essay Scale. *Open Journal of Occupational Therapy*, 4(3), 1–14. Retrieved from http://dx.doi.org/10.15453/2168-6408.1233

10

Writing a
Scholarly Discussion Paper

A discussion paper is a form of refereed journal article in which the author analyzes a professional controversy and argues for a specific resolution. Many authors confuse opinion papers with scholarly discussion papers. A discussion paper analyzes the body of literature about a specific professional controversy and proposes resolutions supported by an analysis of scholarship and research. A discussion paper is a balanced consideration and presentation of all sides of an argument. In contrast, an opinion paper is a one-sided presentation of the author's personal opinions about a professional issue, does not involve rigorous analysis of literature, and bases proposed resolutions on personal agendas rather than a neutral consideration of the literature and stakeholder needs. As with all scholarly writing, the tone of a discussion paper should be neutral. Opinion papers, conversely, convey heightened language and tone to express a particular viewpoint and influence the reader. Opinion papers are appropriate for nonrefereed venues such as newspapers, newsletters, letters to the editor, and magazines. Discussion papers are appropriate for refereed scholarly journals that publish such columns. Authors are encouraged to refer to a journal's author guidelines to determine whether discussion papers are considered for review.

TOPIC SELECTION

Discussion papers address controversies or professional problems whose resolutions will influence the evolution of the profession. A controversy is a dispute about the way in which a problem should be resolved by the profession. Many authors inaccurately think a discussion paper is an exploration of a current topic that may hold importance to the profession but has a clear resolution and is not considered controversial. For example, a discussion of the need to increase the diversity (i.e., race or ethnicity, gender, age) of health care professionals is not a debated controversy and has a clear resolution. The need to increase the diversity of health care professionals is supported by many health care national associations and can be achieved by enhancing the diversity of students

Gutman, S. A. *Journal Article Writing and Publication:
Your Guide to Mastering Clinical Health Care Reporting Standards*
(pp. 127-140). © 2017 Taylor & Francis Group.

entering health care education programs. Examples of currently debated controversies are (a) the degree required for entry-level practice, (b) how multiple health care professions should negotiate overlap in specific areas of practice domain, and (c) the amount and type of activities that can be credited toward continuing education needed to maintain licensure. These examples of controversies are currently debated by health professions and presently have no clear resolution. Authors who wish to write discussion papers that contribute to the literature should select topics of professional controversy. Current topics that have a clear resolution, while enhancing awareness of an issue, do not substantially contribute to the literature and the evolution of a profession.

Examples of Current Topics That Are Not Professional Controversies

- The need to enhance multicultural competence of health care professionals
- The need to enhance health literacy of health care patient information and education
- The need for health care professionals to develop client-centered assessments and interventions that match the health care goals and values of patients

The above topics hold importance to all health professions but are not debated controversies. Arguments against the above are difficult to imagine. Although these topics may not be appropriate for refereed journal articles, they would be appropriate for health magazines, newsletters, and official national association position papers.

Examples of Professional Controversies

- The need for specialty certification within health professions and the criteria to attain and maintain such certification
- Whether physical agent modalities (e.g., ultrasound, electrical stimulation, shortwave diathermy) should be within the practice domain of both occupational and physical therapists
- Whether occupational and physical therapy services should require a physician prescription

These are currently debated controversies having unclear resolutions and would be appropriate discussion paper topics for refereed journal articles.

BASIC CONTENT AND STRUCTURE OF DISCUSSION PAPERS

Discussion papers are approximately 3,000 words in length and have three primary sections. Authors should refer to a specific journal's author guidelines for instructions to write discussion papers. The following sections should be equally weighted and similar in length.

1. Background of the Controversy
2. Presentation of Arguments for and Against the Controversy
3. Directions for Action

Background of the Controversy

Authors should begin discussion papers by describing the controversy and providing background information. The following questions should be answered:

- What is the controversy?
- What is the historical background of the controversy?

- Who are the stakeholders and what are their interests in the controversy and its resolution?
- What is the impact of the controversy on the involved patient population, profession, and larger society?

This section should be based on current literature and use multiple citations.

Presentation of Arguments for and Against the Controversy

In this section authors should present all arguments or viewpoints of the controversial issue using neutral and unbiased language. The following questions should be answered:

- What are the views of all stakeholders?
- What are all sides of the arguments for and against the controversial issue?
- What are proposed resolutions?
- How will all stakeholders be affected by the controversial issue and proposed resolutions?
- What are the authors' views and why? What resolutions do the authors propose and why?

Answers to the above questions should be based on the literature with multiple citations; authors' original ideas and positions, however, do not require citation. It is important that this section be presented as an unbiased and thorough examination of the controversial issue using neutral language.

Directions for Action

In this section, authors should outline the steps that the profession, or professional groups, must take to promote positive resolution of the controversy. These ideas will largely be generated by the authors and do not need to be derived from previous literature and cited. Citations in this section are often minimal. Neutral, unbiased language should be maintained. This section should be written in full narrative paragraphs (as opposed to bulleted phrases).

Tone

As mentioned above, language in discussion papers should be neutral and unbiased. While it is appropriate for opinion papers to use language that is slanted and passionate, authors of scholarly discussion papers to be published in refereed journals must present an impartial analysis and resolution of the controversial issue. While authors are encouraged to use active voice, they should remember that a discussion paper is not an opinion paper based on personal thoughts and perceptions.

EXAMPLE OF THE DEVELOPMENT OF A DISCUSSION PAPER

To illustrate how a discussion paper can be drafted, I will present an editorial that I wrote as editor in chief of the *American Journal of Occupational Therapy*. The editorial was written to introduce a special journal issue about the effectiveness of occupational therapy interventions in mental health practice. Although the paper is written as an editorial, it still possesses many of the components of a discussion paper; however, it is shorter and the arguments are less fully developed. The paper addresses the current state of the occupational therapy profession in the treatment of people with mental health disabilities. Although the profession was once a strongly valued and first-line treatment for people with mental illness, the profession lost its role in mental health care as a result of larger societal historical events, failure to advocate for continued service provision and reimbursement, and failure to adequately provide a description of and evidence for occupational therapy services with this population. The controversy addresses how the profession can regain its once strongly held foothold in the care of youth and adults with mental health disorders.

Gutman, S. A. (2011). Special Issue. Effectiveness of occupational therapy services in mental health practice. *American Journal of Occupational Therapy, 65*(3), 235–237. doi:10.5014/ajot.2011.001339

This article is reprinted with permission from the American Occupational Therapy Association Press.

Effectiveness of Occupational Therapy Services in Mental Health Practice

> The controversy addresses why occupational therapy lost its role in the treatment of people with mental health disorders and how we can regain it. The paper opens with a statement addressing this controversy.

This special issue on the effectiveness of occupational therapy services in mental health practice was compiled in an attempt to further build the evidence supporting the profession's contribution to this practice area. How did we lose our footing in mental health practice when the profession was once considered to be one of the most valued services for people with mental health disorders?

> Here, I begin to outline the historical background of the profession's involvement in mental health care practice.

In the period between World War I and World War II, occupational therapy services were considered to be an essential component of the treatment arsenal for people with psychiatric disorders (Ellsworth, 1983; Gutman, 1995; Wish-Baratz, 1989). Our profession grew out of the Moral Treatment era in the early 19th century—a movement based on the idea that people with psychiatric disorders should be treated humanely and in safe and sanitary environments (Peloquin, 1989; U.S. Department of Health and Human Services, 1999). Providing people with occupations that could engage their minds and interests, and quiet impulsivity and anxiety, even temporarily, was, at that time, considered to be one of the most effective treatments for adults with chronic mental illness (Levine, 1987). Treatment in this period was provided in large state and private institutions where patients were commonly housed for years, often for life (U.S. Department of Health and Human Services, 1999). Discharge was infrequently a consideration. At this time in the profession's history, a majority of occupational therapists were employed in mental health facilities (Quiroga, 1995).

Here, I begin to identify stakeholders (underlined) and their roles in the profession's decline in mental health service provision.

In 1963, <u>Congress</u> passed the Community Mental Health Act, which mandated that treatment of adults with mental illness be provided in the least restrictive setting and support community integration (Ray & Finley, 1994). This act was the impetus for the <u>deinstitutionalization movement</u> in which large state and private mental health facilities closed, and patients were released to community settings—such as group homes—where people were expected to live and receive supportive services (Sharfstein, 2000). In many instances, however, deinstitutionalization outpaced the development of and funding for needed community services, and many former patients became homeless (Accordino, Porter, & Morse, 2001). As treatment of people with mental illness transitioned from large in-patient institutions to the community, occupational therapy positions, like many other mental health care positions, were lost. In the years in which mental health care services transitioned from institution-based to community-based provision, certain health care professions (e.g., <u>psychiatry, psychology, nursing, social work</u>) rebounded and became part of policy-making decisions while occupational therapy did not. Why didn't occupational therapists sufficiently advocate for their role in mental health community integration at this time? <u>Society, insurers,</u> and <u>legislators</u> demanded treatment that could help adults with mental illness to participate as fully as possible in community life and become contributing members of society. Teaching and maintaining self-care and hygiene skills, work skills, medication management, budgeting and bill paying, and home management were services congruent with the profession's domain of concern. Yet, occupational therapy continued to be perceived by health care colleagues and legislators as the provision of crafts to divert the mind (Mosey, 2004). Our health care colleagues and legislators did not understand the relevancy of occupational therapy services, nor did they perceive how such services could be a key element in the community integration of people with mental illness. Why?

Description of historical background and stakeholder interests (underlined) continues in the next paragraph.

In 1975, the Education for All Handicapped Children Act, later becoming Individuals with Disabilities Education Act, was passed. This act mandated that children with special needs receive occupational therapy services in the public school system (U.S. Department of Education, 2007). Many occupational therapists who lost employment in mental health practice transitioned to school-based practice. In the next four decades, the number of occupational therapists working in mental health practice steadily and significantly declined (Stancliff, 1996). Occupational therapy positions that were available in mental health settings remained unfilled for long periods of time and were often eventually filled by other health care professionals or paraprofessionals. Today, health care colleagues, legislators, and society do not commonly associate mental health services with occupational therapy practice. In many states, occupational therapists are no longer considered to be approved and reimbursable providers of mental health services (Swart, 2003; Willmarth, 2005).

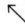

The underlined text states the impact of the controversy on the profession of occupational therapy and larger practice area of mental health care.

In the next paragraph I begin to present arguments addressing how the profession may have undermined its role in mental health care practice. In a full discussion paper, the following section could be separated by a new subheading. Additionally, each argument could be more fully developed.

How did this state of affairs come to exist? Over the last three decades, scholars have pondered this question and have offered the following explanations:

- At the time of transition from large intuitional care to community integration, the profession was neither able to sufficiently advocate for its role in community service provision nor able to flexibly embrace these healthcare changes. Some have argued that it may have been easier for therapists to leave mental health practice and enter school-based therapy than to fight for the profession's role as mental health service provision changed (Mosey, 2004).

- The profession has not been able to sufficiently document the effectiveness of occupational therapy services in mental health practice—not because such services lack effectiveness but because the profession has lacked trained researchers able to carry out intervention outcome studies (Gutman, 2009a). In addition, the majority of research to date has largely focused on the psychometric properties of assessments and basic research describing the experience of disability and the nature of occupation (Case-Smith & Powell, 2008; Gutman, 2008, 2009b).

- A gap may exist between actual clinical practice and the writings that appeared in the profession's literature over the last four decades. Although this gap appears to be narrowing as scholars focus more heavily on evidence-based practice and research, some researchers have argued that the types of topics discussed in our literature have been divorced from the realities of the clinical setting. The profession may not have adequately described and documented its role in mental health practice sufficiently for administrators, legislators, and insurers to understand how occupational therapists help people with chronic mental illness to learn daily life skills needed to function optimally in the community (Rebeiro, 1998).

- The shortage of occupational therapy positions in mental health practice may be mirrored by the larger, national crisis in which mental health services do not share reimbursement parity with physical health services (Buchmueller, Cooper, Jacobson, & Zuvekas, 2007). Occupational therapy students may perceive that mental health practice is not economically feasible, particularly as college education costs have spiraled and students graduate with significantly greater student loan debt than at any other time in the profession's history (Stancliff, 1996).

The views of stakeholders—including occupational therapy practitioners, educators, researchers, and students, as well as patients and legislators—are considered in the above paragraph.

The following paragraph presents directions for action—steps that the profession needs to take in order to rectify the problem. In a full discussion paper, this section could be separated by a subheading, and proposed resolutions could be more fully developed.

While it is likely that all of these factors have contributed in some part to the current occupational therapy mental health care crisis, effective solutions will require coordinated effort between the national association, national foundation, and occupational therapy researchers and practitioners.

- The national association and foundation must be involved in advocacy efforts on a federal and state level and must fund research examining the effect of occupational therapy services in mental health practice.

- The national association should also advocate for government loan forgiveness programs for occupational therapy students who enter mental health practice upon graduation.

- Researchers must examine the effect and cost-efficiency of occupational therapy services used in mental health practice with actual clients.

- Practitioners must be able to advocate for and clearly articulate to administrators how occupational therapy services help clients learn to use the community living skills needed to function as fully as possible in the larger society. Practitioners must also have access to and be able to rely upon a body of research demonstrating the effectiveness of occupational therapy services in mental health practice.

Because this paper was an editorial describing a special journal issue, I used the section below to discuss how the articles in the special issue provide evidence for the effectiveness of occupational therapy services in mental health practice. In a full discussion paper, authors could insert a similar section in which the literature is reviewed to resolve the problem in question.

The seven articles in this special issue offer beginning evidence supporting the effect of occupational therapy mental health services. Three systematic reviews provide evidence for occupational therapy interventions that promote community integration and normative life role participation (Arbesman & Logsdon, 2011), employment and education (Gibson, D'Amico, Jaffe, & Arbesman, 2011), and activity-based interventions (as opposed to verbally based interventions; Bullock & Bannigan, 2011) for people with chronic mental illness. Three intervention studies provide evidence for the positive effect of a life skills program for adults with mental illness at risk for homelessness (Helfrich, Chan, & Sabol, 2011), an occupational time use intervention for people with chronic mental illness (Edgelow & Krupa, 2011), and an occupational goal intervention addressing executive functions of people with schizophrenia (Katz & Keren, 2011). A fourth intervention study reports the effect of an educational DVD intended to enhance therapists' mental health care practices with older adults (Lysack, Lichtenberg, & Schneider, 2011). Lacking from this special issue are studies examining the effect of occupational therapy mental health interventions for children and adolescents.

This final paragraph is the summation and emphasizes the need for the profession to generate research documenting the effectiveness of occupational therapy service with youth and adults with mental health disorders. In a full discussion paper, a subheading (*Summary* or *Conclusion*) could be inserted.

The generation of sufficient research examining the effectiveness of occupational therapy interventions for people with chronic mental illness has been lacking from the profession's literature for too long and has likely contributed to the present mental health care crisis in the profession. Although this special issue alone cannot meet the demand for high-quality, occupational therapy mental health intervention studies, it has at least begun to address the need. The journal will continue to seek intervention studies that examine the effect of occupational therapy interventions for adults and youth with mental health disorders. It is imperative that researchers, practitioners, and the national association and foundation support efforts to produce this needed research and facilitate similar strategies to ensure that the profession regains its former foothold in the mental health practice arena.

REFERENCES

Arbesman, M., & Logsdon, D. W. (2011). Occupational therapy interventions for employment and education for adults with serious mental illness. *American Journal of Occupational Therapy, 65*(3), 238–246. doi:10.5014/ajot.2011.001289

Accordino, M. P., Porter, D. F., & Morse, T. (2001). Deinstitutionalization of persons with severe mental illness: Context and consequences. *Journal of Rehabilitation, 67*(2), 16–21. Retrieved from http://ezproxy.cul.columbia.edu/login?url=http://proquest.umi.com/pqdweb?did=74308446&sid=2 &Fmt=2&clientId=15403&RQT=309&VName=PQD

Buchmueller, T. C., Cooper, P. F., Jacobson, M., & Zuvekas, S. H. (2007). Parity for whom? Exemptions and the extent of state mental health parity legislation. *Health Affairs, 26*(4), w483– w487. doi:10.1377/hlthaff.26.4.w483

Bullock, A., & Bannigan, K. (2011). Activity-based group work in community mental health: A Systematic review. *American Journal of Occupational Therapy, 65*(3), 257–266. doi:10.5014/ ajot.2011.001305

Case-Smith, J., & Powell, C. A. (2008). Research literature in occupational therapy, 2001-2005. *American Journal of Occupational Therapy, 62*, 480–486. doi:10.5014/ajot.62.4.480

Edgelow, M., & Krupa, T. (2011). A randomized controlled pilot study of an occupational time use intervention for people with serious mental illness. *American Journal of Occupational Therapy, 65*(3), 267–276. doi:10.5014/ajot.2011.001313

Ellsworth, P. D. (1983). Army psychiatric occupational therapy: From the past and into the future. *Occupational Therapy in Mental Health, 3*(2), 1–6. doi:10.1300/j004v03n02_01

Gibson, R. W., D'Amico, M., Jaffe, L., & Arbesman, M. (2011). Effectiveness of Occupational therapy interventions for recovery in the areas of community integration and normative life roles for adults with serious mental illness: A systematic review. *American Journal of Occupational Therapy, 65*(3), 247–256. doi:10.5014/ajot.2011.001297

Gutman, S. A. (1995). Influence of the US military and occupational therapy reconstruction aides in World War I on the development of occupational therapy. *American Journal of Occupational Therapy, 49*, 256–262. doi:10.5014/ajot.49.3.256

Gutman, S. A. (2008). From the Desk of the Editor—State of the journal [2008]. *American Journal of Occupational Therapy, 62*, 619–622. doi:10.5014/ajot.62.6.619

Gutman, S. A. (2009a). From the Desk of the Editor—Why haven't we generated sufficient evidence? Part I: Barriers to applied research. *American Journal of Occupational Therapy, 63*, 235–237. doi:10.5014/ajot.63.3.235

Gutman, S. A. (2009b). From the Desk of the Editor—State of the journal 2009. *American Journal of Occupational Therapy, 63*, 667–673. doi:10.5014/ajot.63.6.667

Helfrich, C. A., Chan, D. V., & Sabol, P. (2011). Cognitive predictors of life skill interventions outcomes for adults with mental illness at risk for homelessness. *American Journal of Occupational Therapy, 65*(3), 277–286. doi:10.5014/ajot.2011.001321

Katz, N., & Keren, N. (2011). Effectiveness of Occupational Goal Intervention (OGI) for clients with schizophrenia. *American Journal of Occupational Therapy, 65*(3), 287–296. doi:10.5014/ajot.2011.001347

Levine, R. E. (1987). The influence of the Arts and Crafts movement on the professional status of occupational therapy. *American Journal of Occupational Therapy, 41*, 248–254. doi:10.5014/ajot.41.4.248

Lysack, C., Lichtenberg, P., & Schneider, B. (2011). The effect of a DVD intervention on therapists' mental health practices with older adults. *American Journal of Occupational Therapy, 65*(3), 297–305. doi:10.5014/ajot.2011.001354

Mosey, A. C. (2004). *It's more than a matter of words: How language has affected the occupational therapy profession and what this holds for the future.* Paper presented at the First Anne Cronin Mosey Lectureship, New York University, New York.

Peloquin, S. M. (1989). Moral treatment: Contexts considered. *American Journal of Occupational Therapy, 43,* 537–544. doi:10.5014/ajot.43.8.537

Quiroga, V. A. M. (1995). *Occupational therapy history: The first 30 years, 1900 to 1930.* Bethesda, MD: American Occupational Therapy Association Press.

Ray, C. G., & Finley, J. K. (1994). Did CMHCs fail or succeed? Analysis of the expectations and outcomes of the community mental health movement. *Administration and Policy in Mental Health, 21,* 283–293. doi: 10.1007/BF00709476

Rebeiro, K. L. (1998). Occupation-as-means to mental health: A review of literature, and a call for research. *Canadian Journal of Occupational Therapy, 65,* 12–19. Retrieved from http://www.otworks.com/pdf/OT-mentalhealth.pdf

Sharfstein, S. S. (2000). What happened to community mental health? *Psychiatric Services, 51,* 616–620. Retrieved from http://ps.psychiatryonline.org/cgi/content/short/51/5/616

Stancliff, B. L. (1996). Roundtable. Would you choose mental health OT? *OT Practice, 1*(2), 17–19.

Swart, J. (2003). Capital Briefing. Is an occupational therapist a mental health professional? *OT Practice, 8*(17), 9.

Willmarth, C. (2005). California workers' compensation reform: Implications and strategies. *Work Programs' Special Interest Section Quarterly, 19*(2), 2–4.

Wish-Baratz, S. (1989). Looking Back. Bird T. Baldwin: A holistic scientist in occupational therapy's history. *American Journal of Occupational Therapy, 43,* 257–260. doi:10.5014/ajot.43.4.257

US Department of Education. (2007). *Special Education and Rehabilitative Services. Archived: A 25 Year history of the IDEA.* Retrieved from http://www2.ed.gov/policy /speced/leg/idea/history.html

US Department of Health and Human Services. (1999). *Mental health: A report of the Surgeon General—Executive summary.* Retrieved from http://www.surgeongeneral.gov/library/ mental-health/summary.html

CHECKLIST FOR WRITING A SCHOLARLY DISCUSSION PAPER

- Select a professional controversy.
- Outline the paper using three primary sections:
  1. Background of the Controversy
     - Answer the following questions:
       - What is the controversy?
       - What is the historical background of the controversy?
       - Who are the stakeholders and what are their interests in the controversy and its resolution?
       - What is the impact of the controversy on the involved patient population, profession, and larger society?
     - Use the literature and citations.
     - Keep tone and language neutral.
  2. Arguments For and Against the Controversial Issue
     - The following questions should be answered:
       - What are the views of all stakeholders?
       - What are all sides of the arguments for and against the controversial issue?
       - What are proposed resolutions?
       - How will all stakeholders be affected by the controversial issue and proposed resolutions?
       - What are the authors' views and why? What resolutions do the authors propose and why?
     - Use the literature and citations.
     - Keep tone and language neutral.
  3. Directions for Action
     - Present the steps that the profession, or professional groups, must take to promote positive resolution of the controversy.
     - Because directions for action are based on the authors' ideas, citations in this section will often be minimal.
     - Maintain neutral language and tone.

REFERENCES

American Occupational Therapy Association. (2009). Diverse workforce. Summary of student recruitment activities. Retrieved from http://www.aota.org/en/Practice/Manage/Multicultural/Diverse-workforce.aspx

Gutman, S. A. (2011). Special Issue. Effectiveness of occupational therapy services in mental health practice. *American Journal of Occupational Therapy, 65*(3), 235–237. doi:10.5014/ajot.2011.001339

Turning Academic and Clinical Work Into Publishable Journal Articles

TURNING DOCTORAL WORK INTO JOURNAL MANUSCRIPTS

An increasingly popular model for research doctoral degree programs requires students to develop three research journal articles based on their dissertation. This requirement helps doctoral students transform their dissertation into separate but related journal article manuscripts that can be submitted to various journals. Dissertation committee members, who may be listed as coauthors in the published work, provide guidance regarding the development of the three journal manuscripts. This model helps students transition from the role of doctoral student to academic author.

Most research doctoral degree programs, however, are based on the traditional model in which the student completes novel research and reports the results in a dissertation. Dissertations can often exceed 100 typed pages and are commonly structured by independent chapters that more aptly resemble a book than a research article. The same is frequently true of clinical doctoral theses. Students are commonly expected to develop the skills needed to transform a dissertation or thesis from a 100+ page manuscript consisting of multiple chapters into several 25-page journal manuscripts on their own.

Returning to Your Research Questions

To begin transforming the dissertation or thesis into several research articles, authors should return to their research questions. Commonly, dissertations and theses involve a novel examination of several research questions and subquestions designed to investigate a specific topic. The most efficient way of turning the dissertation or thesis into multiple journal manuscripts is to pull out the primary research questions and structure manuscripts around them.

Gutman, S. A. *Journal Article Writing and Publication: Your Guide to Mastering Clinical Health Care Reporting Standards* (pp. 141-147). © 2017 Taylor & Francis Group.

Let us consider, for example, a doctoral student whose dissertation examined the effect of an intervention designed to help homeless adults transition to supportive housing.

Dissertation research questions consisted of the following:

1. What are the self-identified occupational needs of formerly homeless adults who now reside in supportive housing?

2. How do common physical, cognitive, and mental health problems of this population impact daily function in supportive housing?

3. Can an occupational therapy intervention effectively help formerly homeless adults in supportive housing function better in daily life activities compared to adults in a waitlist control group?

The dissertation was divided into the following chapters based on the three research questions above:

1. Introduction: The State of Homelessness in the United States Today

2. Literature Review

   • Who Becomes Homeless and Why?

   • Types of Supportive Housing for Homeless Adults

   • The Role of Occupational Therapy in the Transition to and Maintenance of Supportive Housing

3. Methods

4. Results

   • Self-Identified Occupational Needs of Formerly Homeless Adults Residing in Supportive Housing

   • Physical, Cognitive, and Mental Health Problems of Formerly Homeless Adults that Impact Daily Function in Supportive Housing

   • Effect of an Occupational Therapy Intervention to Help Formerly Homeless Adults Residing in Supportive Housing to Function Better in Daily Life Activities

5. Discussion

This dissertation was restructured into three journal manuscripts based on the dissertation research questions. Background information about homelessness from the dissertation's introduction and literature review was used in all three articles, but reworded in each manuscript to avoid self-plagiarism and violation of journal copyright regulations.

   • The first manuscript reported the findings yielded from the following dissertation research question: What are the self-identified occupational needs of formerly homeless adults who now reside in supportive housing? In this substudy of the dissertation, the author used qualitative methods to interview seven male and female adults who were homeless for a range of 3 to 5 years to determine their self-perceived occupational needs. The author found that the participants, once housed, led isolated lives but wished to better integrate and participate in community life. Desired occupations included volunteerism, joining supportive housing recreational groups, and obtaining employment. Fear of being in the community and lack of foundational educational skills impeded participants' ability to engage in desired occupations. The author used the manuscript formatting guidelines for a general research study in Chapter 3 to revise this specific dissertation material into a separate, stand-alone manuscript.

   • The second manuscript reported the findings from the following dissertation research question: How do common physical, cognitive, and mental health problems of this population impact daily function in supportive housing? To answer this substudy question, the author used a mixed-method design in which qualitative interviewing was used to understand the types of physical, cognitive, and mental health problems participants perceived as impediments to their daily function in supportive housing. The author also used the Westmead Home Safety Assessment (Clemson, Fitzgerald, & Heard, 1999) to perform an environmental evaluation of the supportive housing environment. Participants commonly reported that memory problems (largely from substance abuse histories and assault) impacted their ability to manage medications and medical appointments and return to school or work. Participants also experienced a range of physical problems—primarily chronic pain—which prevented their participation in community life, hindered their function in the supportive housing apartment, and disrupted sleep. Posttraumatic stress disorder was also experienced by many of the participants, who stated that they had difficulty being in crowds on the subway and city streets and preferred to be alone. The manuscript formatting guidelines for a general research study in Chapter 3 were used to revise this material into a separate, stand-alone manuscript.

- The third manuscript derived from the author's dissertation reported the findings from the following research question: Can an occupational therapy intervention effectively help formerly homeless adults in supportive housing function better in daily life activities compared to adults in a waitlist control group? To answer this question, the author nonrandomly divided her convenience sample into two groups: an intervention group of four participants who received the occupational therapy intervention and a waitlist control group of three participants. The intervention consisted of environmental modifications to the home to enhance function and safety in the bathroom, kitchen, and bedroom. Cognitive compensatory strategies were used to help participants with medication management, medical appointment tracking, and money management. After the 3-month intervention, participants in the intervention group reported enhanced function in the supportive housing environment (e.g., being able to rise from the bed and toilet more easily) and had lowered their incidence of forgetting to take medication or attend medical appointments. Participants in the waitlist control group did not show the same improvement in safety and function. The author used the manuscript formatting guidelines for intervention effectiveness studies in Chapter 4 to revise this material into a separate, stand-alone manuscript.

- A fourth journal article could have reported the details of one participant's intervention experience in a case report format. Using the guidelines for case reports in Chapter 6, the author could have illustrated the characteristics of the intervention by describing the participant's baseline, intervention, and postintervention functional activity status.

When authors develop separate, stand-alone journal manuscripts from their dissertation as novice writers, it is important to seek feedback from seasoned academic writers. If feedback and revision offered by mentors is significant, mentors may be offered coauthorship to ready the manuscript for publication. Working with mentors to develop separate journal articles from the dissertation is a valuable learning experience and can help novice writers learn academic writing skills.

Commonly Made Mistakes in the Transformation of Dissertations and Theses to Journal Articles

One commonly made mistake that novice authors make when transforming their dissertation or thesis into separate journal manuscripts is to submit dissertation chapters without revising them in accordance with reporting standards and journal author guidelines. Sometimes authors cut and paste pieces from the original dissertation without attempting to reformat the work into a cohesive and logically flowing journal manuscript. Authors must remember that the dissertation has distinct requirements and objectives that differ from those of a journal manuscript.

Dissertations and theses are required to adhere to the style guidelines of a specific university rather than a journal. Students sometimes make the mistake of believing that the research procedures and style guidelines taught by their university mentors are the only correct methods and do not consider the need to revise before submitting to a journal. It is imperative to seek the author guidelines of specific journals to which authors wish to submit and revise doctoral work in accordance with those guidelines. It is also critical to use the reporting standards for specific types of research studies to transform doctoral work into publishable journal articles.

It is essential that authors transform their dissertations or theses into publishable journal manuscripts as quickly as possible after the completion of doctoral work. Too often, authors make the mistake of accepting faculty positions or engaging in family and life events, and allow too much time to elapse after doctoral degree completion. Soon the dissertation or thesis becomes abandoned as more time passes and authors become involved in other activities. Failing to transform the dissertation or thesis into two or more journal articles is a lost opportunity because the data have been collected and the research analyzed. Having access to collected and analyzed data that are ready to be developed into one or more journal manuscripts will never occur as readily again.

Turning Doctoral Degree Class Assignments Into Publishable Discussion Papers

Occasionally doctoral students take courses in which they complete paper assignments that they later wish to transform into a publishable discussion paper addressing a professional issue. When doctoral students wish to turn their class paper assignments into discussion papers for publication, it is essential to revise the paper into a journal manuscript that matches a specific journal's publication goals and style guidelines. Some authors make the mistake of submitting paper assignments as originally written or do not read the journal's author guidelines to determine whether a paper topic and format are congruent with the journal's publication objectives. Authors wishing to revise coursework into publishable discussion papers should read Chapter 10, Writing a Scholarly Discussion Paper.

CHECKLIST FOR TURNING
DOCTORAL WORK INTO JOURNAL SUBMISSIONS

- ☐ To transform dissertation and thesis work into journal manuscripts, take the primary research questions and structure manuscripts around them.

- ☐ Although authors can use material from the dissertation or thesis introduction and literature review as background information in multiple journal manuscripts, the wording should be altered in each manuscript to avoid self-plagiarism and copyright violations.

- ☐ Identify the types of research manuscripts (e.g., general research manuscript, intervention effectiveness manuscript, instrument development and testing manuscript, case report manuscript, or discussion paper manuscript) you will develop from the dissertation or thesis and use the reporting standards in this book as formatting guides.

- ☐ Identify journals whose publication objectives correspond to your study and obtain their author guidelines. Use the author guidelines to determine such things as appropriate style guide and limitations on number of references, tables, figures, and words.

- Seek feedback on manuscript drafts from seasoned academic writers. Consider inviting seasoned academic writers to become coauthors to make revisions needed for journal submission readiness.

- Do not submit dissertation or thesis chapters as originally written without making modifications needed for journal submission.

- Do not cut and paste original pieces from the dissertation or thesis without attempting to rewrite the manuscript into a cohesive and logically flowing stand-alone paper. Cutting and pasting pieces from the original doctoral work into a journal manuscript will make the manuscript appear disjointed, poorly organized, and lacking continuity.

- Transform the dissertation or thesis into publishable journal articles as quickly as possible after completing doctoral work. The longer authors wait to publish articles from their doctoral work, the less likely they will be to accomplish this achievement.

- To transform a class assignment into a publishable discussion paper, authors should revise their writing in accordance with the author guidelines of a specific journal to which they wish to submit. Do not submit the assignment as originally written for a specific class. Make sure that the journal to which you wish to submit publishes discussion papers similar to yours.

TURNING CLINICAL DATA INTO POSSIBLE RESEARCH STUDIES

As health care practitioners, we learn to be consumers of research, rather than researchers, in our entry-level programs. Research skills require a set of sophisticated and complex competencies to objectively understand clinical phenomena and assess the effect of interventions designed to treat those phenomena. Research skills are learned in research doctoral programs that require a minimum of 3 years of coursework followed by additional years to complete a novel research study contributing to the profession's body of knowledge. A further year of postdoctoral work as a research assistant in a seasoned researcher's lab is often undertaken to finely hone research skills in a specific area of study.

Retrospective Studies

Clinicians have access to patients and patient databases, and can often formulate fundamental and relevant clinical research questions about evaluation and treatment practices. The collaboration between clinicians and researchers is a vital one needed to ask and answer the most critical questions about clinical practice. Clinicians who wish to participate in research but do not have specific, well-defined research questions should contact health care academic faculty and researchers to determine whether collaborative research can be developed based on the clinical database to which practitioners have access. In this context, a retrospective research study can be designed in which a research question is asked and answered using already collected patient data that will be decoded to protect patient anonymity and confidentiality. For example, a clinician may work with patients who have moderate spasticity in their upper extremities resulting from neurologic insult. A research study could be formulated that examines the effectiveness of two different types of splints. The patient database could be used to examine functional outcomes of similar patients who received splint A compared to splint B.

In another example of the use of retrospectively collected data, a clinician in the school system may work with second graders with handwriting deficits identified by teachers. The database could be used to examine the effectiveness of handwriting interventions that were provided (a) in the classroom in a group format or (b) in one-on-one pullout sessions with the child and therapist.

Although retrospective studies require institutional review board (IRB) approval, they may be easier to conduct than prospective studies because they do not require participant recruitment;

participant and/or guardian consent; and blinding procedures for recruiters, interveners, data collectors, and data analysts. These elements of prospective studies enhance design rigor but are more difficult to implement. Often clinicians who participate in prospective studies do so as data collectors in collaboration with principal investigators who are able to oversee study design formulation, IRB approval, participant recruitment and consent, blinding procedures, intervention fidelity measurement, data analysis, and dissemination of results. Clinicians who wish to participate in prospective studies should contact health care academic faculty and researchers at regional institutions of higher learning to determine whether collaboration is possible.

Case Reports

The reporting of novel intervention through the case report is a form of retrospective research that can be easily accomplished by clinicians who have provided treatment. Because the case report only addresses one patient's treatment experience, it is easier to accomplish than retrospective studies having large databases. In the case report, clinicians have usually provided unique intervention to one patient having positive outcomes. The intervention may show promise of helping more patients with similar clinical conditions, and thus the reported findings are disseminated to the clinical community. For example, a clinician may document the intervention provided to a patient with traumatic brain injury who has significant visual-perceptual deficits. The case report addresses patient history, intervention description, baseline measures, postintervention outcomes, and patient satisfaction. Although Chapter 6 provides details about the formatting necessary for writing a case report manuscript, I recommend that clinicians who are not comfortable with academic journal writing seek mentorship from a seasoned academic writer. An academic writer may be offered coauthorship if he or she significantly contributes to the writing of the final manuscript, which may be necessary for manuscript publication readiness.

CHECKLIST FOR TURNING
CLINICAL DATA INTO POSSIBLE RESEARCH STUDIES

- Determine whether as a clinician you have access to a specific patient database and what type of information is provided in that database (patient demographics, clinical conditions, intervention, outcomes, etc.).
  - Determine whether you have specific clinical questions about evaluation and practice that can be answered through a retrospective examination of your patient database or if a seasoned researcher and faculty member can help you formulate clinical questions.
  - Contact and meet with seasoned researchers to refine research questions, develop study procedures, seek IRB approval, implement study, collect data, analyze data, and report written results using an appropriate manuscript reporting standard format.
- Determine whether as a clinician you have a unique patient case that can be turned into a case report for publication.
  - Determine whether the intervention provided is novel or if the patient's clinical condition has not been previously addressed by your profession and documented in the literature.
  - Make sure that you have collected baseline and postintervention measurements using standardized instruments.
  - If you do not feel comfortable with the academic writing skills needed to construct a case report manuscript for publication (as described in Chapter 6), seek help from a seasoned

academic researcher or faculty member. If this professional assumes a significant portion of the writing, coauthorship should be negotiated.

REFERENCE

Clemson, L., Fitzgerald, M. H., & Heard, R. (1999). Content validity of an assessment tool to identify home fall hazards: The Westmead Home Safety Assessment. *British Journal of Occupational Therapy, 62*(4), 171–179.

12

Ethical Considerations in Publication

Just as there are ethical issues concerning research misconduct (e.g., mistreatment of participants, failure to gain participant consent and institutional review board approval, and fraudulent data analysis and reporting), ethical issues also pertain to publication misconduct. Publication misconduct is the unethical management of manuscript preparation, submission, and publication. This section addresses issues such as plagiarism, dual submissions, inappropriate authorship, copyright violation, and failure to disclose conflict of interest. Some of these activities are erroneously committed by authors due to lack of knowledge. Understanding common acts of publication misconduct will help you avoid these in the publication process.

AUTHORSHIP

Authorship is the assignment of ownership to a piece of written scholarship. Authorship should be decided in the early stages of a research project, when roles and activities are defined and assigned. The definition and assignment of roles and activities should be recorded in writing and disseminated to all involved parties. The dissemination process of the written record should request that authors respond to any inconsistencies or inaccuracies by a specified date and that receipt of the document (such as through email) serves as an acknowledgement of agreement unless otherwise specified in writing.

Authorship order should also be decided in the early stages of the project in accordance with the rigor of contributions made to the project by each identified author. First authorship is assigned to the researcher who contributes most to the study design, research implementation, and manuscript writing and preparation. Subsequent authorship is then assigned in accordance with each researcher's contributions. When initial authorship identification and order are decided, it must be acknowledged and understood by all authors that authorship may change if researchers cannot fulfill their specified roles or cannot contribute at the level to which they first committed.

Gutman, S. A. *Journal Article Writing and Publication: Your Guide to Mastering Clinical Health Care Reporting Standards* (pp. 149-155). © 2017 Taylor & Francis Group.

The granting of authorship should be made to researchers who contribute substantially to the conception and design of the study, data collection and analysis activities, and manuscript preparation and submission. Honorary authors (i.e., authors who do not contribute to the study and manuscript preparation but who are listed as authors) and ghost authors (i.e., authors who substantially contribute to study conduction and manuscript writing but are not acknowledged) are examples of inappropriate research practices that prevent full transparency and accountability to the scientific community and public. Honorary authors are often used to increase a study's credibility and impact. Ghost authors are commonly used when manufacturers (such as pharmaceutical or medical equipment companies) carry out a study to demonstrate the effect of their products but falsely list academicians as authors. The practice of ghost writing in health care publication also occurs when seasoned mentors design and/or write significant sections of doctoral student dissertations but are not credited. Both instances of ghost authorship involve falsification of intellectual property and prevent full transparency of and accountability for a research study design and findings.

Research doctoral students who are in the process of turning their original doctoral research into published articles should take responsibility for first authorship but also credit mentors with either authorship or acknowledgment depending on the level of the mentors' contributions. Entry-level health care students who implement a faculty member's research study as part of degree requirements may or may not be considered as authors on a submitted research paper. If students worked on some component of the faculty member's research and helped to collect or analyze data without making any other significant contribution to the study design, implementation, or manuscript preparation, students should be acknowledged for their contribution rather than credited with authorship. If students substantially contributed to multiple components of the design, data collection, analysis, and/or manuscript preparation, student authorship should be considered.

PLAGIARISM

Piracy is the misappropriation of ideas, data, or work as one's own, instead of obtaining permission from or acknowledging the original authors (Committee on Publication Ethics, 2014). Plagiarism is a form of piracy that specifically involves the misappropriation of written work (including images, tables, and figures) as one's own, rather than obtaining permission from or acknowledging the rightful authors. Plagiarism in journal publication is considered to be an egregious violation of intellectual property rights and truthfulness of ownership. Many acts of plagiarism are unintentional and occur as a result of poor research practices. For example, when reviewing the literature on a specific topic, some authors may copy passages from published articles without making notes indicating that the material has been copied verbatim. They may later use that verbatim material because they forgot that the passage was copied and believed it to be their own words. Today many journals use plagiarism check software programs that can identify plagiarized work in the review process.

Many authors have called for greater leniency of plagiarism definitions with regard to their own work. The publishing world and academia now recognize that authors should be able to use and rework their ideas in multiple publications (Columbia University Copyright Advisory Office, 2009a). Although verbatim sentences and paragraphs from previously published articles should not be used in subsequent manuscripts, authors are able to use similarly written language and ideas to discuss their work in multiple published articles without being accused of plagiarism and without violating copyright laws. Use of the same data set in multiple publications without disclosure, however, is considered to be a form of research misconduct.

Many authors also serve as reviewers for professional journals. Reviewers must maintain high ethical standards and confidentiality and recuse themselves from manuscript reviews that may present conflicts of interest. Reviewers are commonly asked to review papers whose topics match the reviewer's area of expertise. In such cases, it is unethical for reviewers to use data and information obtained from a manuscript review without crediting the original source. Cases have been disclosed in which reviewers who were exposed to new ideas and data as part of the manuscript review process, plagiarized such data and ideas in their own work without crediting the original authors, and sabotaged the authors' manuscript causing rejection. When reviewers act unethically, they are removed from journal review boards, can lose their academic positions, and are often informally blackballed from their profession.

TRANSPARENT REPORTING OF DATA, METHODS, AND CONFLICT OF INTEREST

Transparency in research reporting is critical to maintain credibility and the trust of the scientific community and public. In past decades the journal publishing world endorsed a third-person writing style that obscured critical details about researcher roles and study methods that could potentially bias results. Today, journal writing endorses a first-person writing style and requires authors to disclose the roles and activities of all researchers in a study so that readers can evaluate the existence of possible bias. The journal world's adoption of formal reporting standards for clinical studies has also facilitated the transparent reporting of research methods and findings.

Key elements of a research manuscript must be reported transparently. Researchers must clearly report the following:

- Whether institutional review board (or ethics committee) approval was obtained or exempted
- Whether participant consent was obtained for adults; parental or guardian consent and child assent were obtained for minors
- Whether consent was obtained for patients whose data were used in a case report
- Whether any adverse events occurred in the study that impacted results or held implications for the use of the intervention with patients
- Whether the full set of data was used as opposed to data from only those participants who were able to tolerate the testing conditions and/or intervention and completed the study
- Whether missing data exist (the protocol for handling missing data must be reported)
- Whether researchers were blinded to group assignment and study purpose
- Whether the profession, training, and blinding procedures of the interveners and data collectors were appropriate for study intent
- Whether interveners were also data collectors
- Whether results were discussed only in the context of literature that supported the researchers' findings while ignoring contrary evidence

Additionally, authors must declare all conflicts of interest. A conflict of interest is a circumstance in which a person derives benefit from a particular situation or event, usually at the expense of others. In journal publication, authors may hold personal interest and derive benefit from the findings of a study. Authors' research may be funded by a source that holds a vested interest in a particular outcome. For example, a researcher's study may be funded by a self-care equipment company that will benefit from studies demonstrating the effectiveness of their products with patients. A researcher may earn monetary derivatives from a newly developed clinical product, such as an edema wrap, and hold a vested interest in studies demonstrating product effectiveness. A researcher may have a family member who owns stock in a motorized mobility equipment company and be involved in patient satisfaction research with such equipment. Authors are required to declare such conflicts of interest and the role of funders in research.

Manuscript reviewers must declare conflicts of interest that may exist before accepting review solicitations. For example, reviewers who engage in similar research as that of the manuscript authors and compete for scarce grant funding with that research team should declare a conflict of interest and recuse themselves from review. Reviewers who believe they can identify the authors of a research manuscript with whom they hold professional disagreements should also recuse themselves from review. In general, if as a reviewer you cannot remove your emotions from the review process and produce a neutrally written review—for personal or professional reasons—you should recuse yourself as a reviewer for that paper. Similarly, many journals allow authors to identify reviewers with conflicting interests and request that such reviewers not be solicited for manuscript review.

DUAL SUBMISSION, PIECEMEAL PUBLICATION, AND REANALYSIS OF DATA

Dual submission (also referred to as simultaneous or multiple submission) is the concurrent submission of the same paper to different journals without disclosing that the paper is being reviewed by more than one journal. When authors submit a paper to a journal they are commonly asked to confirm that the manuscript is original and has not been submitted elsewhere. Dual submission constitutes an ethical breach of the review process because the same research paper cannot be published by multiple journals without the journals' knowledge and agreement of dual copyright status. If authors have submitted a paper to a specific journal and then wish to submit to another instead, the editor of the first journal must be contacted and the manuscript withdrawn from review.

Piecemeal submission is the unnecessary division of one research study into two or more papers to increase publications. If a research study can be published as one paper and fit journal word count limitations, authors should aim to publish the study in its entirety in one journal article. The only instances that warrant multiple publication of the components of one research study occur when the research components can stand alone, when the authors cannot fit the entire elements of a research study into a single manuscript's page length requirement, and when the material is better organized through the presentation of several papers. An example would be a psychometric measurement study of a specific instrument. If multiple psychometric properties (such as inter-rater reliability, test-retest reliability, content validity, and convergent validity) have been assessed in one study but cannot be adequately presented in one paper, authors may elect to publish results in two papers. When publishing the results of one study in separate papers, authors should always disclose that results were derived from one study and cite the original paper describing the study.

Reanalysis of data is the use of a published data set to answer different research questions presented in a subsequent manuscript. A paper in which published data are reanalyzed to explore new research questions is legitimate when the data set can truly reveal new and important findings and when the authors disclose that the data set has been previously analyzed and published. When already published data sets are reexamined to yield information about the relationships among variables and do not significantly contribute important knowledge to the profession and society, the research appears disingenuous and authors appear to be "fishing" for additional publications. In reanalysis of data, authors must always clearly disclose that the data have been derived from an already published data set and cite the original journal article.

COPYRIGHT

Copyright is the assignment of legal ownership rights to a given work. While authorship denotes the creators of a work, copyright grants owners the ability to publish and reuse the work. It is common for journals to require manuscript authors to sign a copyright agreement transferring ownership rights to the journal. Although the authors maintain their authorship status, they generally lose control over publication of the article. Many academic organizations have challenged the journal publishing world to modify outdated copyright agreements so that manuscript authors have the right to use their work in future educational and scholarly endeavors, control the future use of their work, and facilitate access of their work by members of the scholarly community (Columbia University Copyright Advisory Office, 2009b; Securing a Hybrid Environment for Research Preservation and Access, 2006).

The most common rights that authors should seek in journal copyright agreements regarding the future use of their work include the following:

- The right to reproduce and distribute the work in teaching
- The right to reprint sections of the work in future articles or books
- The right to reuse sections of the work in the creation of related or derivative work (e.g., journal articles, books, and professional presentations)
- The right to be credited as author of original work that has been released in another form
- The right to post journal articles (in preprint or postprint form) to university digital repositories
- The right to post federally funded journal article research (in preprint or postprint form) to federal digital repositories in accordance with governmental policies

Authors should never transfer copyright of their assessments, clinical guidelines, photographs, illustrations, or unique figures that they will likely wish to use again in publication and education. Instead, authors should maintain copyright of these items and grant the journal permission for one-time printing. The U.S. Copyright Act automatically grants copyright ownership of original work without requiring any action from authors such as copyright registration; however, copyright registration is recommended for items that are potentially marketable, such as clinical assessments and instruments and continuing education course content (United States Copyright Office, 2009). Authors should make sure that the journal identifies the authors as the copyright owners of a specific item in a note published beneath the item. Maintaining copyright of specific materials eliminates situations in which authors lose control of these items and are forced to pay for and seek permission to use their own work.

Anytime that authors wish to reprint already published materials whose copyright is owned by a journal (such as tables, figures, and assessments), authors must obtain permission from that journal. As mentioned in previous sections of this book, quotations should be avoided in scholarly writing with the following exceptions: a quotation from a historical or legal document, a specific definition accepted by the scientific community whose meaning would change if the exact wording were altered, and specific statements made by participants in qualitative studies. If you quote a passage from a published source that is 50 words or more, many journals require permission from the copyright owner.

CHECKLIST FOR TRANSPARENT AND ETHICAL PUBLICATION PREPARATION AND SUBMISSION

- ☐ Decide who will receive authorship and in what order early in the project.
- ☐ Record authorship designation and order in written form (all authors should maintain a copy).
- ☐ To receive authorship, all authors should have made substantial contributions to the manuscript.
- ☐ Submit the final manuscript version to a plagiarism check software program to avoid inadvertent violations of copyright.
- ☐ Authors who use their own previously published material in future work should not use verbatim sentences; ideas and similar language can be used.
- ☐ Use a first-person writing style and disclose the roles and activities of all researchers in the study so that readers can evaluate the existence of possible bias.
- ☐ Indicate whether institutional review board (or ethics committee) approval was obtained or exempted.
- ☐ Indicate whether participant consent was obtained for adults and assent for minors.
- ☐ Indicate whether consent was obtained for patients whose data were used in a case report.
- ☐ Report the occurrence of any adverse events in the study that may have impacted results or hold implications for the use of the assessment or intervention with patients.
- ☐ Indicate whether the full set of data was used as opposed to data from only those participants who were able to tolerate the testing conditions and/or intervention and completed the study.
- ☐ Indicate whether missing data exist and describe the protocol for handling missing data.
- ☐ Indicate whether researchers were blinded to group assignment and study purpose.
- ☐ Describe the profession, training, and blinding procedures of the interveners and data collectors (in an intervention effectiveness manuscript).
- ☐ Disclose if interveners were also data collectors (in an intervention effectiveness manuscript).
- ☐ Be clear that results were discussed in the full context of literature rather than only literature supporting the findings.
- ☐ All authors must declare any conflicts of interest and describe the funder's role in the research.
- ☐ Submit the manuscript to one journal at a time; indicate that the manuscript is original and is not being reviewed simultaneously by another journal.
- ☐ If the manuscript is based on a larger study or is a component of another study, disclose this to readers and cite the original study.
- ☐ Indicate if the manuscript is a reanalysis of previously published data and cite the original study.
- ☐ All authors should sign the copyright release form and maintain a copy.
- ☐ Make sure that the copyright agreement allows for basic author rights to reuse one's own work in education and derivative work and to post work to open-access repositories.
- ☐ Do not transfer copyright of assessments, clinical guidelines, and unique images if you intend to use these again in other publications. Instead grant the journal one-time permission to reprint.
- ☐ Make sure to obtain permission to reprint any materials owned by another source.

REFERENCES

Committee on Publication Ethics. (2014). Principles of transparency and best practice in scholarly publishing. Retrieved from http://publicationethics.org/files/Principles_of_Transparency_and_Best_Practice_in_Scholarly_Publishing.pdf

Columbia University Copyright Advisory Office. (2009a). What is fair use? Retrieved from http://copyright.columbia.edu/copyright/fair-use/what-is-fair-use/

Columbia University Copyright Advisory Office. (2009b). Overview. Retrieved from http://copyright.columbia.edu/copyright/copyright-ownership/overview/

Securing a Hybrid Environment for Research Preservation and Access. (2006). Authors and open access. Retrieved from http://www.sherpa.ac.uk/guidance/authors.html#funderrurles

United States Copyright Office. (2009). Copyright basics. Retrieved from http://www.copyright.gov/circs/circ01.pdf

Index

Printed in the United States
by Baker & Taylor Publisher Services